TITANIUM ALLOYS FOR BIOMEDICAL DEVELOPMENT AND APPLICATIONS

TITANIUM ALLOYS FOR BIOMEDICAL DEVELOPMENT AND APPLICATIONS

DESIGN, MICROSTRUCTURE, PROPERTIES, AND APPLICATION

Zhentao Yu
Jinan University, Guangzhou, P.R. China

Elsevier
Radarweg 29, PO Box 211, 1000 AE Amsterdam, Netherlands
The Boulevard, Langford Lane, Kidlington, Oxford OX5 1GB, United Kingdom
50 Hampshire Street, 5th Floor, Cambridge, MA 02139, United States

Copyright © 2022 Elsevier Inc. All rights reserved.

No part of this publication may be reproduced or transmitted in any form or by any means, electronic or mechanical, including photocopying, recording, or any information storage and retrieval system, without permission in writing from the publisher. Details on how to seek permission, further information about the Publisher's permissions policies and our arrangements with organizations such as the Copyright Clearance Center and the Copyright Licensing Agency, can be found at our website: www.elsevier.com/permissions.

This book and the individual contributions contained in it are protected under copyright by the Publisher (other than as may be noted herein).

Notices

Knowledge and best practice in this field are constantly changing. As new research and experience broaden our understanding, changes in research methods, professional practices, or medical treatment may become necessary.

Practitioners and researchers must always rely on their own experience and knowledge in evaluating and using any information, methods, compounds, or experiments described herein. In using such information or methods they should be mindful of their own safety and the safety of others, including parties for whom they have a professional responsibility.

To the fullest extent of the law, neither the Publisher nor the authors, contributors, or editors, assume any liability for any injury and/or damage to persons or property as a matter of products liability, negligence or otherwise, or from any use or operation of any methods, products, instructions, or ideas contained in the material herein.

British Library Cataloguing-in-Publication Data
A catalogue record for this book is available from the British Library

Library of Congress Cataloging-in-Publication Data
A catalog record for this book is available from the Library of Congress

ISBN: 978-0-12-823927-8

For Information on all Elsevier publications
visit our website at https://www.elsevier.com/books-and-journals

Publisher: Matthew Deans
Acquisitions Editor: Christina Gifford
Editorial Project Manager: John Leonard
Production Project Manager: Prasanna Kalyanaraman
Cover Designer: Victoria Pearson

Typeset by MPS Limited, Chennai, India

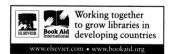

Contents

List of contributors	vii
Preface	ix

1. Overview of the development and application of biomedical metal materials — 1

1.1 Biomedical stainless steels	1
1.2 Biomedical CoCr alloys	5
1.3 Biomedical shape memory alloys	9
1.4 Biomedical noble metals	11
1.5 Biomedical refractory metals	13
1.6 Ti and its alloys	17
1.7 Degradable metals	19
References	24

2. Design and physical metallurgy of biomedical β-Ti alloys — 27

2.1 Overview of design methods of biomedical Ti alloys	27
2.2 Overview of composition design of biomedical Ti alloys	32
2.3 Overview of the design and development of typical biomedical β-Ti alloys	34
2.4 Smelting and physical metallurgical properties of typical β-Ti alloys	39
2.5 Design and physical metallurgical properties of novel TLM alloy	45
References	51

3. Processing, heat treatment, microstructure, and property evolution of TLM alloy — 55

3.1 Overview of processing and heat treatment of β-Ti alloys	55
3.2 Billets and semifinished products of TLM alloy	56
3.3 Plates and strips of TLM alloy	58
3.4 Bars and rods of TLM alloy	65
3.5 Tubes of TLM alloy	71
3.6 TLM alloy products with special specifications	77
3.7 TLM alloy foils	83
References	88

4. Biological and mechanical evaluation of TLM alloy — 91

4.1 Biological evaluation of TLM alloy	91

4.2 Biomechanical compatibility of TLM alloy	109
References	123

5. Surface modification and functionalization of TLM alloy — 125

5.1 Surface modification of Ti alloys	125
5.2 Surface functionalization of Ti alloys	128
5.3 Surface dealloying of TLM alloy	134
5.4 Bioactive coatings on TLM alloy	137
5.5 Wear-resistant coatings on TLM alloy	144
5.6 Anticoagulant coatings on TLM alloy	148
5.7 Antimicrobial coatings on TLM alloy	153
References	159

6. Development and application of TLM alloy for the replacement and repair of surgical implants — 163

6.1 Development and application of traditional Ti implants	163
6.2 Design and novel manufacture of Ti implants	165
6.3 Implants for orthopedics and trauma repair	170
6.4 Implants for joint repair and replacement	174
6.5 Implants for oral and maxillofacial repair and replacement of TLM alloy	185
6.6 Medical devices of TLM alloy for spine repair	195
References	196

7. Development and application of TLM alloy for treatment of soft tissue with minimally invasive surgery — 199

7.1 Development and application survey of minimally invasive devices	199
7.2 Design and manufacture survey of interventional devices	201
7.3 Coronary stents of TLM alloy	204
7.4 Nonvascular stents and related devices of TLM alloy	212
7.5 Shell of brain and heart active devices of TLM alloy	216
7.6 Other minimally invasive and interventional devices of TLM alloy	222
Reference	223

Index — **227**

List of contributors

Lei Jing Northwest Institute for Non-Ferrous Metal Research, Xi'an, P.R. China

Xiqun Ma Northwest Institute for Non-Ferrous Metal Research, Xi'an, P.R. China

Sen Yu Northwest Institute for Non-Ferrous Metal Research, Xi'an, P.R. China

Zhentao Yu Jinan University, Guangzhou, P.R. China

Preface

New materials are the basis and forerunner of new technological revolutions, and the development and application of these materials are important milestones of human social civilization and material progress. Biomedical materials are used mainly to diagnose, treat, or replace human tissues and organs or to improve their functions. They are high-tech materials with advanced structures or functions that are widely applicable and have high economic value. They cannot be replaced by drugs and have become one of the most vigorous research fields in materials science.

Epoch-making medical devices, such as titanium hip joints, titanium dental implants, CoCr vascular stents, and titanium artificial hearts, have saved the lives of patients and improved their quality of life. Among all the biomedical metal materials, such as Ti alloys, CoCr alloys, TiNi alloys, and 316L and 317L stainless steels, the advanced biomedical titanium and its alloys have been or are becoming the main and key raw materials for surgical implants and minimally invasive interventional devices.

Since the beginning of the 21st century, in order to continuously improve and enhance the functional diversity, biological safety, biomechanical compatibility, and long-term application of biomedical titanium alloy materials, research on the alloy design, novel material development, processing and preparation, microstructure and property evaluation, and product application of these materials has been deepening and becoming a research hotspot in the field of new biomaterials in the world. This book consists of seven chapters, focusing primarily on alloy design, physical metallurgy, materials processing, microstructure and mechanical properties, surface modification, advanced manufacturing, and clinical research of novel biomedical beta-type TLM titanium alloy. The book also offers a comprehensive and systematic introduction into the research and development achievements of the author's research group in the past 18 years.

The first chapter describes the latest research progress of alloy design, typical microstructure, mechanical properties, and clinical applications of commonly used medical metals (stainless steels, cobalt–chromium alloys, titanium alloys, shape memory alloys, etc.) and degradable metals (magnesium alloys, zinc alloys, etc.).

In the second chapter the alloy design, selection of alloy elements, process and preparation, and physical metallurgy of the new generation of metastabilized beta-type TLM titanium alloys are introduced, and the main mechanical properties of the typical beta-type titanium alloys that have been developed at home and abroad are summarized.

The third chapter introduces the research on the cold and hot processing, heat treatment, related typical microstructure, and mechanical properties of the raw materials of plates, rods, and tubes made of novel TLM alloys and introduces the advanced manufacturing methods and typical microstructure and mechanical properties of the tubes in small-diameter and thin-wall-thickness foils and strips and extrafine wires of TLM titanium alloy.

The fourth chapter introduces the biological evaluation (hemocompatibility, cytotoxicity, genetic toxicity, skin and oral stimulation, bone implantation, etc.) of the novel TLM alloy material, and the results of research into biomechanical compatibility of TLM alloy, including superelasticity and shape memory effects, high- and low-cycle fatigue behavior, and wear resistance.

The fifth chapter introduces the research and evaluation on surface processing and modification treatments, surface functional coatings, and their biocompatibility with body tissues (cells) of novel TLM titanium alloy, which aims to improve the biological activity, wear resistance, and anticoagulant ability of titanium alloy, in order to endow the surface multifunctioning of titanium alloy materials.

The sixth chapter introduces the research and development of novel TLM titanium alloy materials in the field of surgical implants, focusing on the structural design, finite element numerical simulation, advanced manufacturing, and performance evaluation of some typical devices for repairing human hard tissue, such as dental implants and artificial hip joints.

The seventh chapter introduces the research and development of TLM titanium alloy special materials that are used in typical minimally invasive interventional products and active medical devices, focusing on the structural design, processing, and manufacturing process of some typical devices, such as vascular stents and cardiac pacemakers, and their related performance evaluation.

The book should be helpful to researchers, teachers, technicians, and graduate students, who are engaged in basic and applied research, development, and education with regard to biomedical metals by introducing some new materials, new technologies, new methods, and new products of medical titanium alloys. The book is also expected to contribute to our understanding of the research and development of new biomaterials and medical devices, especially to achieve the following purposes:

1. To deepen the understanding of alloy design methods and physical metallurgical properties control of new medical metal materials such as titanium alloys.
2. To grasp the basic principles and key technologies of processing, preparation, heat treatment, microstructure and mechanical properties, and adjustment and control of basic raw materials and special materials of medical titanium alloys.
3. By comprehensively introducing the biological and biomechanical properties, functional coating, and new surface modification technology of the novel TLM titanium alloy materials, to strengthen the understanding of the application of this new type of titanium alloy material in custom design functionality and the long-term effects of various implantable and interventional medical devices.
4. By introducing the simulation design, advanced manufacturing process, and application performance of some typical medical devices of the novel TLM titanium alloy, to promote the application of these high-end products in a variety of biomedical engineering fields.

The literature referred to in this book is derived mainly from the previous research results of my group from Northwest Institute for Nonferrous Metal Research (NIN). The major contributors involved in the compilation of this book are Professor Sen Yu (Chapters 5–7), Professor Xiqun Ma (Chapters 2 and 3). Engineer, and Dr. Lei Jing (Chapters 1 and 4). The other colleagues who participated in the survey and collation of the published literature are Senior Engineer Yafeng Zhang (Sections 3.5, 3.6, 7.3, and 7.4), Senior Engineer Jun Cheng (Sections 1.6, 2.5, 2.6, and 3.1), Senior Engineer Binbin Wen (Sections 6.3, 6.4, 6.5, and 7.5), Professor Jinlong Niu (Sections 2.3 and 2.7), Engineer Hanyuan Liu (Sections 1.2 and 1.3), Engineer Chang Wang (Sections 1.7 (Chapter 1 and 4 and 7.1), Professor Yusheng Zhang (Section 5.5), Senior Engineer Wangtu Huo (Section 5.5), Engineer Qi Shen (Section 7.2), Engineer Xi Zhao (Section 2.1), and Engineer Wei Zhang (Section 5.5). The other colleagues who participated in the survey and collation of the published literature and who work in Xi'an Jiuzhou Biomaterials Co., Ltd. are Professor Jianye Han (Sections 6.4 and 6.5), Senior Engineer Qiang HuangFu (Sections 3.5, 3.6, 7.1, and 7.3), Senior Engineer Sibo Yuan (Section 6.5), Engineer Hui Liu (Sections 6.3 and 6.4), and Engineer Xiaoyan Shi (Sections 6.1 and 7.1).

The study of surface bioactivity modification of novel TLM titanium alloy materials in this book (Section 5.4) has been supported by Professor Yong Han from Xi'an Jiaotong University. The biosafety evaluation of novel TLM titanium alloy materials in this book has also been supported by Professor Yumei Zhang (Sections 4.1.6, 4.1.7, and 4.1.8) and Professor Minghua Zhang (Section 4.1.9) from PLA Air Force Military Medical University and Professor Xiaohong Li (Sections 4.1.2, 4.1.3, and 4.1.4) and Professor Kunzheng Wang (Sections 4.1.5 and 4.1.9) from Xi'an Jiaotong University.

My colleagues and graduate students from NIN and Jinan University assisted me in the English translation and proofreading of this book. Professor ZengXiang Fu from Northwestern Polytechnical University and Associate Professor Weihong Jin and Dr. Baisong Guo from Jinan University put in a lot of effort into the English review and proofreading of this book. My doctoral and master students, Lan Wang, Xiaojun Dai, Longchao He, and Yunhao Xu from NIN and Qingyun Fu, Mingcheng Feng, Wenqi Liang, Jiaxin Huang, and Yue Wu from Jinan University took part in the English translation of this book.

Finally, I am grateful to the above people for their strong support during the book editing and publishing. In addition, as a result of my limited knowledge and writing ability, there might be some errors and omissions in the book. I sincerely welcome criticism, guidance, and correction by readers.

Zhentao Yu[1,2]

[1]*Biomedical Materials Technology Research Center, Institute of Advanced Wear & Corrosion Resistant and Functional Materials, Jinan University, Guangzhou, P.R. China* [2]*Biomaterials Research Center, Northwest Institute for Non-Ferrous Metal Research, Xi'an, P.R. China*

CHAPTER 1

Overview of the development and application of biomedical metal materials

1.1 Biomedical stainless steels

1.1.1 Overview of biomedical stainless steels

Biomedical stainless steel has good biocompatibility, mechanical properties, and corrosion resistance as well as excellent processing and forming capabilities, and it has a low cost. Therefore it is a class of metal materials that have been widely used in medical devices and equipment.

Because of the lack of intergranular corrosion resistance and stress corrosion resistance of traditional industrial stainless steel, biomedical stainless steel materials mainly incorporate austenitic stainless steel with the best corrosion resistance to reduce the dissolution of potentially harmful metal ions in the alloy, such as nickel and chromium ions. This puts forward higher requirements for the composition regulation of medical stainless steel. Medical stainless steel usually requires strict control of Ni and Cr content and low impurity element content, and the size of nonmetallic inclusions should not exceed grade 1.5 (fine series) and grade 1 (coarse series). In addition, the carbon content in the alloy must not exceed 0.03% to improve its intergranular corrosion resistance [1]. The detailed chemical compositions are listed in Table 1.1.

However, the Ni element that is used to stabilize the austenite phase in stainless steel tends to cause some tissue reactions and other problems when it dissolves, such as contact dermatitis and eczema, and it may cause cancer and may even cause restenosis after the cardiovascular stent to some extent, which is life threatening. Therefore domestic

TABLE 1.1 Comparison of chemical compositions of typical medical stainless steel materials (wt.%).

Material	C	Cr	Ni	Mn	Mo	Si	S	P
06Cr19Ni13Mo3 (S31708) 317	≤0.080	18.0–20.0	11.0–15.0	≤2.00	3.0–4.0	≤1.00	≤0.030	≤0.045
022Cr19Ni13Mo3 (S31703) 317L	≤0.030	18.0–20.0	11.0–15.0	≤2.00	3.0–4.0	≤1.00	≤0.030	≤0.045
06Cr17Ni12Mo2 (S31608) 316	≤0.080	16.0–18.0	10.0–14.0	≤2.00	2.0–3.0	≤1.00	≤0.030	≤0.045
022Cr17Ni12Mo2 (S31603) 316L	≤0.030	16.0–18.0	10.0–14.0	≤2.00	2.0–3.0	≤1.00	≤0.030	≤0.045

Source: data from GB/T 1220–2007 Stainless Steel Bars, Standardization Administration of China.

and foreign research institutions have begun to develop a series of new biomedical stainless steels such as low-nickel or nickel-free austenitic stainless steel and antibacterial stainless steel to meet the increasing requirements of the medical and health field.

1.1.2 Nickel-free austenitic stainless steels

Ni mainly plays a role in stabilizing the austenite phase in austenitic stainless steel. Therefore it is necessary to add a new nontoxic austenite stable element to replace Ni to develop Ni-free austenitic stainless steel. Nitrogen is an ideal austenite stabilizing element with a low cost. It has a strong strengthening effect as an interstitial atom, which can significantly increase the strength of stainless steel without reducing its plasticity. Because the Ni element was replaced with a relatively high content of N to stabilize the austenitic structure of stainless steel, nickel-free stainless steel has also been called high-nitrogen nickel-free (HNNF) stainless steel [2], which has been the most widely used.

For example, 0.9 wt.% N element in BIOSSN stainless steel can give it the plasticity and twofold strength of 316L stainless steel [1,3]. The Fe21Cr22Mn1Mo1N HNNF stainless steel developed in the United States has been put into the US medical market to replace CrNi series stainless steel. China has also made important achievements in this regard and has developed Fe17Cr14Mn2Mo(0.45−0.7)N biomedical HNNF austenitic stainless steel with excellent comprehensive properties, such as high strength, fatigue resistance and excellent wear resistance [3]. The mechanical properties, such as tensile strength (R_m), yield strength (R_p), elongation (A), and area reduction (Z), of HNNF stainless steel are shown in Table 1.2.

TABLE 1.2 Mechanical properties of HNNF stainless steel.

Material	R_p (MPa)	R_m (MPa)	A (%)	Z (%)	A_{kV} (J/cm^2)	H_v
316L (solution)	225	555	64	72	290	164
Co62Cr28Mo6 (solution)	492	1013	19	24	33	318
HNNF stainless steel (solution)	537	884	52	71	193	262
HNNF stainless steel (10% cold deformation)	857	1008	36	73	–	316
HNNF stainless steel (20% cold deformation)	1041	1105	30	70	–	350
HNNF stainless steel (30% cold deformation)	1175	1215	24	68	–	380

Source: data from GB/T 1220−2007 Stainless Steel Bars, Standardization Administration of China.

1.1.3 Antibacterial stainless steels

With the development of society and the improvement of people's health awareness, the threat from the spread of bacteria has attracted increasing attention. Accordingly, people have put forward higher requirements for the antibacterial properties of biomedical stainless steel. Humans have long realized that metal ions such as silver and copper ions have strong antibacterial effects [4,5]. The antibacterial effects of metal ions are as follows: Hg > Ag > Cd > Cu > Zn > Fe > Ni. The antibacterial effect of the specific alloy depends on whether there are enough active particles of the element on the alloy surface. For example, Fe and Ni have certain antibacterial functions; however, it is difficult to show their antibacterial functions because the passivation layer or oxide layer forms easily on the metal surface.

Although many metals have antibacterial functions, not all elements are suitable for use as antibacterial elements for comprehensive safety and antibacterial properties reasons. At present, the most commonly used antibacterial elements are Cu and Ag. It has been found that that after adding Cu element to stainless steel, a uniformly dispersed and stable ε-Cu phase will be formed in the stainless steel matrix, which can provide a long-lasting and stable antibacterial effect.

Hong et al. [6] studied the effect of copper content and aging treatment on SUS 304 austenitic stainless steel and found that the residual ferrite content in as-cast SUS 304 steel decreased with the increase of Cu content and that the addition of Cu inhibited the formation of martensite induced by strain. Corrosion tests show that the pitting potential decreases with the increase of Cu content in SUS 304 steel. The results of the antibacterial test show that the addition of an appropriate amount of Cu (2 wt.%) can give SUS 304 stainless steel excellent antibacterial properties. When the added amount of Cu exceeds 3.5 wt.%, even if the aging time is as short as 30 minutes, the antibacterial rate can reach 99.99%. However, the amount of added Cu should not exceed 3.5 wt.% to ensure that the Cu-containing SUS 304 steel can achieve a balance between formability, corrosion resistance, and antibacterial properties. Chen and Thouas [7] found that dissolved Cu^{2+} plays a major antibacterial role in antibacterial stainless steel, which led to the collapse of some lipopolysaccharide patches on the cell surface, thus changing the permeability and physiological function of the extracellular membrane, providing a structural basis for the antibacterial effect of Cu^{2+} on microorganisms.

1.1.4 Application

According to a previous study [1], when the Ni content exceeds 12 wt.%, single-phase austenite can be obtained, and Cr can form a

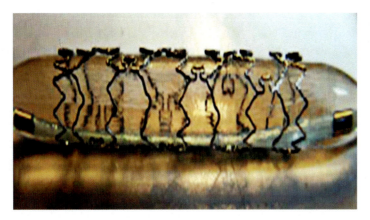

FIGURE 1.1 Coronary stent of HNNF stainless steel.

chromium oxide passivation film to improve corrosion resistance. As the N content increases, the HNNF austenitic stainless steel has better anticoagulant performance. Therefore the new biomedical stainless steel not only can be used to make artificial joints, spinal internal fixation systems, and fracture internal fixation devices, such as bone plates, bone screws, and surgical tools, but also can be utilized in cardiovascular systems, such as in artificial heart valves and intravascular stents. A typical coronary stent made from HNNF austenitic stainless steel is shown in Fig. 1.1. It can also be used for dental crowns, dental orthopedic wires, ophthalmic sutures, artificial eye wires, orbital fillings, and other medical devices.

1.2 Biomedical CoCr alloys

1.2.1 Overview of CoCr alloys

The first application research of CoCr alloys in surgical implant can be dated to the 1930s, when they were made as cast parts and then forged alloys. The casting, extrusion, and forging conditions have a significant effect on the corrosion resistance and mechanical properties of the alloy. Generally speaking, casting tend to produce coarse grains, grain boundary separation, porosity, and shrinkage in CoCr alloys. Although casting alloys are superior to noncasting alloys in terms of wear resistance, pitting resistance, and crevice corrosion resistance, they are inferior to forged alloys in terms of fatigue strength and fracture toughness. Therefore the use of precision casting can eliminate the structural defects of the alloys and also improve their mechanical properties. The use of forging, extrusion, rolling, drawing, and other hot pressure processing methods can further ameliorate the as-cast structure of the material and achieve better mechanical properties [7]. In addition, with the development of three-dimensional (3D) printing technology, the use of 3D to prepare CoCr alloy products is a new method that has high processing speed and strong customization and can be effectively applied in treating bone defects and dentistry.

Co-based alloys are generally CoCr alloys, of which there are two basic types: CoCrMo alloy and CoNiCrMo alloy. Six types of alloys have been included in medical standards. The CoCr–Mo alloy has an austenitic structure, which can be produced by forging or casting, but it is very difficult by cold deformation. Its mechanical properties and corrosion resistance are better than those of stainless steel, making it a relatively good biomedical metal material. Forged Co-based alloys are used mainly to make replacement prostheses for knee and hip joints. The American Society for Testing and Materials recommends four CoCr alloys that can be used in surgical implants: forged CoCrMo (F76), forged CoCrWNi (F90), forged CoNiCrMo (F562), and forged CoNiCrMoWFe (F563), in which F76, F90, and F562 have been widely used in the manufacture of surgical implants. A comparison of the mechanical properties of different metal implant materials is shown in Table 1.3.

Owing to the relatively high content of Cr in CoCr alloys, Cr spontaneously forms an inert oxide layer (Cr_2O_3) in the human environment, so the corrosion resistance of CoCr alloys is better than that of stainless steel. As in stainless steel, Cr, Mo, and Ni all have corrosion resistance. Tungsten (W) is added to increase solid solution strengthening and control the distribution and size of carbides, but it will also reduce the corrosion resistance and corrosion fatigue strength of CoCr-based alloys. The dissolution of Co and Ni from CoCr alloys will cause cell and tissue necrosis. Co, Ni, and Cr can also cause allergic skin reactions, of which Co has the greatest impact. Therefore it is of the utmost importance to strictly control the phase structure, grain size, and ion dissolution limit of CoCr alloys.

1.2.2 Typical microstructure and properties of CoCr alloys

CoCr alloys are generally composed of solid solution–strengthened austenite matrix and carbides distributed in the matrix. The type and content of precipitated phases are controlled by regulating the heat treatment processes to strengthen the matrix. CoCr alloys have low stacking fault energy, leading to the formation of a large number of annealing twins after annealing [8]. Li et al. [9] studied the microstructure evolution of biomedical L605 alloy during the process of multipass thermomechanical processing (TMP), indicating

TABLE 1.3 Comparison of mechanical properties among different CoCr alloys.

Materials	Brand	ISO	ASTM	R_m (MPa)	R_p (MPa)	A (%)	Condition
Co28Cr6Mo	CoCrMo	5832–4	F75	655	450	8	Cast
Co20Cr15W10Ni	L605	5832–5	F90	1250	760	15	Hard
Co19Cr17Ni14Fe 7Mo1.5Mn	Grade 2 Phynox	5823–7	F1058	1170–2240	690–1725	1–17	Hard + age
Co20Cr20Ni5Fe 3.5Mo3.5W2Ti	Syncoben	5832–8	F653	1310	1172	12	Hard
Co28Cr6Mo	Wrought CoCrMo Alloy 2	5832–12	F1537	1000	700	12	Hard
Co28Cr6Mo	Wrought CoCrMo Alloy 1	5823–12	F1537	897	517	20	Annealed
Co20Cr15Ni15Fe 7Mo2Mn	Grade 1 Elgiloy	5823–7	F1058	1860–2275	1240–1450	–	Hard + age
Co35Ni20Cr10Mo	MP35N	5832–6	F562	1207	1000	10	Hard
18Cr14Ni2.5Mo	Wrought stainless Steel	5832–1	F138/ 139	490–800	190	40	
				860–1100	690	12	Annealed hard

that after 5 passes of TMP treatment, the grains can be remarkably refined, and a bimodal grain microstructure composed of fine grains (3 μm) and coarse grains (4−16 μm) can be formed. Such a bimodal grain microstructure provides superior mechanical properties with a tensile strength of 1197−1304 MPa, a yield strength of 593−738 MPa, and a uniform elongation of 54.7%−61.1%.

Studies have shown that when the concentration of Cu^{2+} is lower than 500 mm, Cu ions can promote the proliferation of human venous endothelial cells but have an inhibitory effect on the proliferation of arterial smooth muscle cells. Wang et al. [10] and others have studied the effect of the addition of Cu (1−4 wt.%) on the structure, corrosion, mechanical properties, and cytotoxicity of L-605 alloy, aiming to develop a new type of biological functional alloy. The results shown that dendrite segregation occurs in all L-605 alloys with different Cu contents during the casting process, and the addition of copper reduces the corrosion resistance of the alloy, slightly reduces the microhardness of the material, and has a limited effects on the compression performance of the material. CCK8 results shown that L-605 Cu alloy has good cell viability, and the addition of Cu does not cause cytotoxicity.

1.2.3 Typical application of CoCr alloys

Although the Ni content of L-605 is lower than that of 316L stainless steel, sensitive reactions induced by Ni may also occur. Although its mechanical properties are similar to that of CoCrMo alloy, its mechanical properties are twice as high as that of CoCrMo alloy under the condition of cold working deformation of 44%, and the stress corrosion cracking resistance in aqueous solution is also improved. In the work-hardened state, L-605 alloy is still nonmagnetic. Therefore L-605 alloy is commonly used for cardiovascular stents, and its annealed state can be used as a surgical fixation suture. MP35N alloy has very high tensile properties in the work-hardened state and the work-hardened aging state, which has almost the highest mechanical properties among all implanted metal materials. Therefore MP35N is widely used to produce artificial joints, pacemaker electrode wires, stylets, urinary catheters, and orthopedic wires.

In general, compared with stainless steel, CoCr-based alloys have higher strength, more stable passivation film, and better corrosion resistance and wear resistance. Therefore they are more suitable for manufacturing surgical implants in the body for long-term service that need to bear high loads and have high wear and corrosion resistance, such as artificial joints, vascular stents, and dental crowns. Typical medical devices made from CrCo-based alloys are shown in Fig. 1.2.

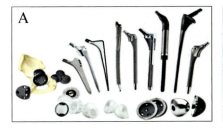 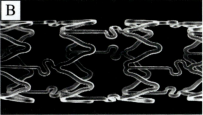

FIGURE 1.2 Typical medical devices of CrCo alloys. (A) Joint prostheses. (B) Stent.

1.3 Biomedical shape memory alloys

1.3.1 Overview of shape memory alloys

Shape memory alloy refers to a type of metal material that can be restored to its original shape and size after a proper thermodynamic process, that is, a type of metal material developed by the principle of reversible martensitic phase transformation. Since the discovery of shape memory phenomenon in the 1960s, more than 20 kinds of memory alloys have been studied around the world and have been widely used. At present, the most widely used memory alloy is TiNi (or NiTi) shape memory alloy [11].

Ni−Ti shape memory alloy has shape memory characteristics and superelasticity in the phase transition zone. At low temperatures (around 0°C) it has a monoclinic crystal phase, which is soft and deformable. When the alloy is heated to a high temperature, it becomes a cubic crystal phase and immediately returns to its original shape and produce a continuous soft restoring force. At this time, the material is hard and elastic, which can be useful in orthopedics or support. The memory recovery temperature of the alloy is close to the temperature of human body (36°C ± 2°C), Because it exhibits good biocompatibility, corrosion resistance, and abrasion resistance, this metal material is called a new functional material in the 21st century [12].

1.3.2 Typical composition and brand of shape memory alloys

NiTi shape memory alloy is an alloy with 54.5−57.0 wt.% Ni. The chemical composition of NiTi shape memory alloy has a significant effect on the phase transition temperature (PTT). For NiTi binary system shape memory alloys, the PTT will decrease by about 10°C for every 0.1% increase in Ni content, which can be controlled by adjusting the Ni content. However, when the Ni content is too high (>51%, atomic fraction), the alloy precipitates Ni-rich compounds such as $TiNi_2$ and $TiNi_3$,

TABLE 1.4 The typical plate, rod, and wire products of NiTi memory alloy.

Material types	Grade	PTT (A_f/°C)	Standard
Rod, wire	NiTi−01/NiTi−02	20−40	ASTM F2063−12/GB 24627−2009
	NiTi−ss	45−90	
	TN3/TNC	5−15	
	NiTi−ss/NiTi−yy	−30 to 20	
	NiTiCu	33 ± 3	
	NiTiNb	As−Ms ≤ 5	
	NiTi−ss	As−Ms < 150	
Plate	NiTi−01/NiTi−02	20−40	
	NiTi−ss	45−90	
	NiTi−yy	5−15	

which reduces Ni content in matrix, resulting in an increase in the PTT and brittleness of the alloy. The addition of a third element to the TiNi alloy will also significantly affect the PTT. For example, adding V, Cr, Mn, or Al to replace Ti or adding Co or Fe to replace Ni can lower the PTT. The detailed PTTs of different NiTi memory alloys are shown in Table 1.4.

1.3.3 Typical application of NiTi shape memory alloys

At present, NiTi shape memory alloys are used mainly for cardiovascular and cerebrovascular and nerve interventional treatments, such as cardiovascular stents, cerebrovascular stents, and peripheral vascular stents for laryngotracheal, esophageal, and urethral stenosis, as well as percutaneous transluminal coronary angioplasty catheter shafts, nerve terminal area stent catheters, internal and mirror inspection delivery systems. In the fields of artificial joint replacement, spinal repair, trauma surgery, and sports medicine, NiTi shape memory alloys can be used for artificial joints, spinal correction devices, patella claws, patellar collectors, bone plates, sternum fixators, embracing devices, and tension hooks. In the field of oral cavity and dentistry, these alloys can be used for dental orthopedics and dental surgical treatment tools, such as dental arch wires, dental memory fixators, and root canal files. In the fields of cardiovascular surgery, general surgery, urology, gastroenterology, gastrointestinal otolaryngology, and other fields, the alloys can be used for surgical accessories for endoscopic examination and laparoscopic surgery, such as valve regulators, tissue retractors, surgical tools, and catheters.

1.4 Biomedical noble metals

Noble metals have good corrosion resistance and ductility as well as good biocompatibility and physiological nontoxicity. Therefore they are widely used in the medical field and have broad application prospects in dentistry, acupuncture, implantable electronic devices, precious metal drugs, and medical biosensors [13].

1.4.1 Dental materials

Gold is the first metal to be used in dental materials. As early as 2000 years ago, ancient people used gold to fix or fill teeth. Since the dental gold alloys are used mostly to make jewelry or gold coins, such as AuAgCu, Au10Cu, and AuPtPd, these alloys are easy to form rough segregated grains during casting and solidification. Sometimes the alloy loses luster in the environment, so people try to improve its corrosion resistance by adding other alloying elements. For example, adding a small amount of Ru, Os, or Ir to the Au−Pt−Pd alloy can refine the as-cast structure and increase its strength. Adding a certain amount of Pt, Pd, Zn, and other elements to Au−10Cu alloy can give it better anticorrosion and antidarkness abilities and can present different colors, providing more choices for patients with different oral esthetic needs [13−15].

Since 1968, to reduce the cost of materials, a series of dental gold alloys with low gold content have been studied, including precious metal casting alloys and porcelain fused to metal alloys. In addition, owing to their price advantage, nonprecious metals also occupy a place in the dental market, gradually forming the three pillars of gold alloys, palladium-based alloys, and nonprecious metal alloys. The common compositions of noble alloys are shown in Table 1.5.

1.4.2 Acupuncture materials

Acupuncture and moxibustion are important practices in traditional Chinese medicine. They are not only unique in their methods, but also have remarkable curative effects. Acupuncture has been developed and applied in more than 100 countries, such as the United States, France, and Germany. Acupuncture needles mainly include gold needles, silver needles, and hard needles. The hard needles are mainly made of stainless steel. Because of the low hardness of pure gold and silver, these elements not suitable to be used as a needle, so the hardness must be improved by alloying. At present, the commonly used gold needles are made of 10K, 12K, 14K, and 18K gold, of which 14K gold is the most

TABLE 1.5 AuAgCu alloy composition.

Color	Types	Composition (wt.%)					
		Au	Ag	Cu	Pd	Pt	Zn
Yellow	Soft gold	79–92.5	3–12	2–4.5	<0.5	<0.5	<0.5
Yellow	Medium hardness gold	75–78	12–14.5	7–10	1–4	<1	0.5
Yellow	Hard gold	62–78	8–26	8–11	2–4	<3	1
Yellow		60–71.5	4.5–20	11–16	<5	<8.5	1–2
White	Hard gold	65–70	7–12	6–10	10–12	<4	1–2
Yellow white		60–65	10–15	9–12	6–10	4–8	1–2
White		28–30	25–30	20–25	15–20	3–7	0.5–1.7

Source: data from Y. Wang, Q. Cao, Z. Jia, J. Zheng, Application and development of precious metals in the field of medicine, Rare Metal Materials and Engineering 43 (2014) 165–170.

widely used. Because of the discoloration of silver needles, it is necessary to simultaneously improve their corrosion resistance during alloying. Among the commonly used silver needles, Ag–Pd silver needles have the best corrosion resistance, but their cost is higher. AgSn and AgSnIn alloys have lower cost but poor ductility, while AgCuZn has lower cost and better overall performance.

1.4.3 Medicinal precious metals

Because of the special properties of precious metals, such as antiinflammatory and sterilization, they are widely used in the pharmaceutical industry. The precious metals that have been used to make medicines include gold, silver, platinum, and osmium. In China the use of gold medicine to treat diseases has a long history, which can be traced back to 2500 BCE. Europeans have also used gold medicine to treat depression, fainting, fever, epilepsy, and other diseases. The organic compounds of gold have antiinflammatory effects, and the oral medicine anuranofin, which was developed in 1985, peaked the development of gold medicine [16]. As an oral medicine for treating arthritis, it has many excellent properties that outcompete the injection type. It also has an inhibitory effect on lymphoma and is expected to be a potential anticancer drug.

Silver is a bactericidal metal that is inferior only to mercury. Ag^+ has a strong bactericidal effect with very little consumption. Generally, it can sterilize at a level of 1×10^{-6} mol L^{-1}. In ancient times, people discovered that silverware has a certain anticorrosive and fresh-keeping function. Since the 1990s research and development of silver sterilization materials have drawn great attention. People take advantage of the bactericidal and antibacterial properties of Ag$^+$ to prepare materials with bactericidal functions, such as medical device cleaning fluids, bactericidal bandages, the gauze. Some organic silver compound antibacterial agents can also be used to treat local infections, syphilis, and other diseases.

Platinum drugs are also commonly used precious metal drugs. In the middle of the 18th century, platinum medicine was used to treat syphilis and rheumatism, which aroused people's interest in platinum medicine. In the 1970s, Professor Luxembourg in the United States first reported that cisplatin has broad-spectrum anticancer activity, opening up a new field of anticancer drug research [17].

1.4.4 Surgical materials

Because of their excellent corrosion resistance and biocompatibility, precious metals such as gold and silver are widely used as surgical implant materials. For example, Ag alloy can be used as a craniomaxillofacial substitute material in brain surgery. Silver amalgam cement can be used for orthopedic repair surgery, and high-purity Au membrane is used as ear tympanic membrane repair material. In cancer radiotherapy, implanting Pt-coated Ir wire or wire mesh can shield healthy tissues from radiation damage.

1.5 Biomedical refractory metals

1.5.1 Overview of biomedical refractory metals

Biomedical refractory metals mainly include tantalum (Ta), zirconium (Zr), hafnium (Hf), niobium (Nb), tungsten (W), molybdenum (Mo), and vanadium (V). The common characteristics of these metals are high density, high melting point, high hardness, strong corrosion resistance, good chemical stability, and relatively high price. Therefore they are used mainly as alloy addition elements of stainless steel, cobalt–chromium alloy and titanium (Ti) alloy and thus are usually not used alone as biomedical metal materials. Ti (1–60 wt.%) Zr is a new type of medical alloy that is suitable for the design and development of dental implants, denture brackets, and other dental products. The TiNb

(1−45 wt.%) and TiTa (1−45 wt.%) alloys can be used for orthopedic implants, such as artificial joints [18].

Ta has high stability and good biocompatibility, wear resistance, and corrosion resistance and has no adverse effects on the human body, making it an ideal material for surgical implants. Since the 1940s, Ta material has been widely applied in skull defect repair, joint prosthesis, and other medical devices. It has also been used to produce pacemakers, vascular clips, joint prostheses, and metal wire, sheet, or net used for nerve repair. [19]. In addition, Ta is known as a biophilic metal while the elastic modulus E (186−191 GPa) of the densified pure tantalum is significantly higher than that of the cortical bone tissue (10−30 GPa). The stress shielding problem caused by the modulus E mismatch between artificial implants and host bones will cause the bone resorption around the implant to be greater than the bone formation and at the same time delay the formation of the callus, resulting in a series of complications, such as loosening or fracture of the implant, and finally leading to implant failure.

The use of tantalum porous structure has been found to simulate that of bone tissue and can reduce the elastic modulus of metal implants, thus achieving a good biomechanical match between the implant and the bone tissue. Compared with dense metal Ta, porous Ta materials have a 3D porous microstructure, which increases the contact surface area between the implant and bone tissue. Moreover, the nanoporous microstructure has a huge impact on the proliferation of osteoblasts, and its rough surface can absorb more macromolecules, which facilitate the adhesion and growth of osteoblasts and greatly improve the osseointegration and reconstruction capabilities of the implants and bone tissue [20].

1.5.2 Preparation and evaluation of porous tantalum

Although porous Ta has obvious advantages, its extremely high melting point and easy reaction with oxygen pose a new challenge for the preparation of porous tantalum. Porous Ta is a metal similar to foam or sponge, which was originally developed by the U.S. company Implex. At present, the preparation processes of porous Ta proposed by domestic and foreign scholars mainly include the vapor deposition method, organic foam impregnation method, powder sintering method, and 3D printing method [21].

Currently, vapor deposition is the most widely used method for preparing porous tantalum. The general process is as follows: First prepare an organic framework, then deposit Ta vapor on the framework, and finally remove the framework to obtain porous metallic tantalum. The

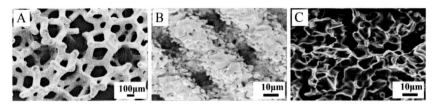

FIGURE 1.3 Scanning electron microscopic images of porous Ta obtained by different preparation methods. (A) Chemical vapor deposition. (B) Powder metallurgy. (C) 3D printing.

porous Ta prepared by this method has a purity of up to 99%, a pore size of 400–600 μm, and a porosity of 75%–85%. The organic foam impregnation method involves immersing the organic foam in the tantalum powder slurry and then preparing porous Ta by vacuum sintering. The pore size is 300–500 μm, and the porosity is about 60%. Although its porosity is low, the porous tantalum prepared by this method has mechanical properties similar to those of natural bone. The porous tantalum prepared by powder sintering has a porosity of 75% and a pore size of 250–300 μm, but this method is prone to produce residual adhesive or organic slurry, and the residue after sintering is toxic and difficult to remove. The 3D printing method is flexible for preparing porous tantalum, providing a new way to control the density and pore size of porous tantalum, and can be used to prepare porous tantalum with special pore structure. The microstructures of porous tantalum prepared by varied approaches are shown in Fig. 1.3.

The pore structure, pore size, and porosity of porous tantalum have an important influence on its mechanical properties and biological activity. Luo [22] prepared porous tantalum scaffolds with different pore sizes and porosities by 3D printing. According to mouse bone marrow stromal cell culture experiments, it was found that too large or too small pore size and porosity are unfavorable for promoting cell adhesion and proliferation and also not conducive to the formation of new bone and the initial stability of the bone implant interface. Porous tantalum scaffolds with a pore size range of 400–600 μm with a porosity of 75% and a pore size range of 600–800 μm with a porosity of 85% have obvious advantages in the process of inducing osteogenic differentiation of cells, and macroporous stents are more likely to act by upregulating the expression of vascular-related factors. Tsao et al. [23] implanted hundreds of prostheses in 98 patients, showing that the hip survival rate of Steinberg stage II patients was 72.5% at 48 months after surgery. The average Harris hip score increased by 20 points, and satisfactory treatment was achieved. In addition, patients implanted with porous tantalum implants such as tibial plateau prosthesis, patella prosthesis, and spinal fusion device, all performed well in postoperative bone healing.

1.5.3 Porous tantalum application

Porous tantalum has broad prospects in clinical applications, and its product promotion and application are closely related to its production process. For example, porous tantalum surgical implants prepared by vapor deposition methods are mainly used for noncustomized prostheses, such as conventional bone nails, bone plates, bone rods, and patches. 3D printing technology is used mainly for mass preparation of personalized porous tantalum prostheses, such as oral implants and intervertebral fusion cages.

Porous implants can be produced rapidly by using advanced processing technologies, such as vapor deposition and additive manufacturing, which are more in line with the pathological and physiological characteristics of patients. Zimmer's first commercially available porous tantalum material (trabecular metal) prepared by vapor deposition has been used in the repair of human cortical bone and cancellous bone [24]. The Chongqing Runze company of China has prepared porous tantalum materials with good performance by reverse mold pore forming and high-temperature and high-vacuum sintering, which have entered clinical evaluation [25]. Currently, the tantalum products, including integrated acetabular cups, dental implants, femoral head support rods, tibial plateau prostheses and tibial cone-shaped fillers, patella prostheses, spinal fusion devices, bone repair patches, bone plates, and bone nails, have been promoted and applied in the field of global medical devices. Two typical devices made of porous tantalum are shown in Fig. 1.4.

In the medical field, Ta metal has many other applications besides prosthetic implants. For example, a metal Ta coating has been prepared on the surface of Ti alloy, glassy carbon, and polymer, which not only can improve the corrosion resistance and biocompatibility of the material, but also can reduce the cost by taking advantage of the low cost

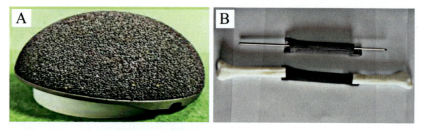

FIGURE 1.4 The clinical application of porous Ta. (A) Standardized porous Ta acetabular cup. (B) Bone defect fibula prosthesis. *Source: data from K. Yang, H. Tang, J. Wang, G. Yang, N. Liu, L. Jia, et al., Research progress of standardized and additive manufacturing of personalized porous tantalum implants. Hot Working Technology 46 (2017) 5−8; L. Yang, F. Wang, Application of medical 3D printing porous tantalum in orthopedics, Journal of the Third Military Medical University 41 (2019) 1859−1866.*

and easy processing of the base material. Such an approach can greatly broaden the application area of metal tantalum [26].

In addition, Ta mesh and Ta sheet can be used to repair muscle or bone defect tissue. Medical Ta silk sutures can be used not only for sutures of tendons, fascia, bones, and nerve fibers, but also for fixing and cerclage of teeth or bones. Through clinical follow-up interviews, it has been found that 94% of fracture patients treated with Ta wire cerclage internal fixation have no complications after surgery, and the treatment effect is also good, demonstrating that the application of porous tantalum as a prosthetic implant is safe and effective.

1.6 Ti and its alloys

In the 1950s and 1960s, stainless steel and cobalt−chromium alloys were widely used. In the late 1970s the two-phase Ti alloy Ti6A14V with medium and high strength began to attract attention and quickly gained popularity in the medical field. Compared with traditional medical metal materials, such as stainless steel and CoCrMo alloy, Ti and Ti alloy have more comprehensive mechanical properties, low elastic modulus, better corrosion resistance, and better biocompatibility and have gradually become the preferred materials in medical fields such as for use in surgical implants.

The development of biomedical Ti and its alloys can be divided into three eras. The first era is represented by commercial pure Ti (CP−Ti, α type) and Ti6A14V ($\alpha + \beta$ type), and the second era is represented by new $\alpha + \beta$ alloys of Ti5A12.5Fe and Ti6A17Nb. The third era features the research and development of novel β Ti alloys with better biocompatibility and lower modulus of elasticity [18].

1.6.1 The first generation of biomedical Ti alloys

In the late 1940s, Ti was first confirmed to be nontoxic through animal experiments. In 1951, CP−Ti was used to manufacture bone plates and screws, but CP−Ti has low strength and poor wear resistance, which limits its application in parts of the body with large stress bearing. At present, it is used mainly for oral restoration and bone replacement for parts with small stress bearing. In contrast, Ti6Al4V has higher strength and better processing properties. It was originally designed for aerospace applications and was widely used as surgical repair materials in the late 1970s in hip joints and knee joints. Ti6A14V ELI (low clearance) alloy has good biocompatibility, corrosion resistance, and mechanical properties. It is the most widely used surgical implant material in clinical practice. Ti3A12.5V is also clinically used as a replacement material for femur and tibia. However, this type of alloy contains potentially toxic aluminum and vanadium. Vanadium is considered to be toxic to organisms and is more toxic than Ni and Cr. It accumulates in the bones, liver, kidneys, spleen, and other organs, and its phosphate is related to the biochemical metabolism and acts by affecting the ATPase of Na^+, K^+, Ca^+, and H^+. Aluminum also has potential toxicity. Its harm to organisms is caused by the accumulation of aluminum salt in the body, thus causing organ damage. Al can also cause symptoms such as osteomalacia, anemia, and neurological disorders [18].

1.6.2 The second generation of biomedical Ti alloys

To avoid the potential toxicity of V, two new $\alpha + \beta$ type biomedical Ti alloys were developed in Europe in the mid-1980s: Ti5Al2.5Fe (developed in Germany) and Ti6Al7Nb (developed in Switzerland). In 1985 the Swiss company Sulzer used forged Ti6Al7Nb alloy to manufacture hip joint handles and was approved for registration. This type of alloy replaces the toxic element V with nontoxic elements such as Nb and Fe, eliminating the toxic side effects of V on the human body. Compared with CP−Ti, their strength is increased by about 2 times, their wear resistance is better, and their mechanical properties are similar to those of Ti6Al4V. However, they still contain Al, and the elastic modulus is still high, 4−10 times higher than that of compact bone. This will lead to a mismatch of elastic modulus between the artificial prosthesis and bone tissue, causing the load not to be well transmitted from the implant to the adjacent bone tissue and thus causing the stress shielding phenomenon, resulting in bone resorption around the implant and eventually leading to the loosening or fracture of the implant.

1.6.3 The third generation of biomedical Ti alloys

In the early 1990s, on the basis of the d electronic alloy design theory proposed by Japanese scholars, researchers in the United States and Japan began to use nontoxic elements such as Nb, Ta, Zr, Mo, and Sn to replace V and Al, and firstly developed a series of new generation of medical β-type Ti alloys that were nontoxic and had low elastic modulus [18].

Ti13Nb13Z alloy with the addition of nontoxic elements Nb and Zr was developed by Smith & Nephew Richards in the mid to late 1990s. This alloy not only has a lower modulus of elasticity (79 GPa) than CP−Ti (105 GPa) and Ti6Al4V (110 GPa), but also has better biocompatibility, becoming the first novel β−type medical Ti alloy to be included in the ISO standard. Later, researchers in the United States developed some novel β-type biomedical alloys, such as Ti12Mo6Zr2Fe (TMZF), Ti−15Mo, Ti16Nb10Hf,

1.7 Degradable metals

Ti15Mo3Nb3O, TIMETAL 21SRx and Ti−35Nb−5Ta−7Zr. The elastic modulus of Ti35Nb5Ta7Zr alloy is very low, only 55 GPa. A novel β-type Ti alloy Ti29Nb13Ta4.6Zr was developed by Niinomi of Tohoku University in Japan [28]. This alloy has an elastic modulus close to that of human bones and good biological and mechanical properties. To improve its fatigue performance and achieve low cost, researchers in Japan also developed Ti15Zr4Ta4Nb0.2Pd0.2O0.05N, Ti15Sn4Nb2Ta0.2Pd0.05O0.004N, and other alloys, which are interstitial solid solution strengthened by adding trace oxygen and nitrogen elements. In 2003, Saito et al. in Japan developed a new set of metastable β-type Ti alloys composed of IVB and V group elements, which have several functional characteristics, such as low elastic modulus, exceptionally high strength, elasticity, and plasticity, and constant elasticity, and were called gum metal [27].

Since the 1980s, researchers in China have been engaged in the research and application of Ti and its alloys in the medical field, especially in orthopedics, and have successfully developed TiNi shape memory alloys, including Ti5Al2.5Fe, Ti6Al7Nb, and Ti2.5Al2.5Mo2.5Zr (TAMZ). Since 2000, Chinese researchers have begun to develop a new generation of β-type Ti alloys, the most representative of which are the Ti3Zr2Sn3Mo25Nb (TLM), Ti15Nb5Zr3Mo (TLE), and Ti10Mo6Zr4Sn3Nb alloys developed by Zhentao Yu's research team of the Northwest Institute for Nonferrous Metal Research (NIN) [29−31] and the Ti2448 (Ti24Nb4Zr7.6Sn) alloy designed and developed by the Institute of Metals, Chinese Academy of Sciences [32]. These novel metastable β-type Ti alloys have good biocompatibility, high strength, and low elastic modulus and are especially suitable for the repair and replacement of various surgical implants, such as artificial joints, dental implants, and internal fixation systems. The mechanical properties of some typical medical Ti alloy materials are shown in Table 1.6.

Although the new third-generation β-type biomedical Ti alloy has clear superiority over other materials, it still has some defects. For example, its elastic modulus is still slightly higher than that of human bone, and its abrasion resistance in the biological environment is poor. In addition, refractory elements such as Nb, Ta, and Hf, which are often added to the alloy, have high density and a high melting point and are expensive. It can be seen that further research and development are needed to find more ideal and cost-effective medical Ti alloys.

1.7 Degradable metals

Since the 1990s the research hotspot of biomedical materials has transferred from biostable materials to degradable or absorbent materials. These are a class of materials that can be completely degraded after being implanted in organisms, and the degradation products can be

TABLE 1.6 Mechanical properties of some typical newly developed Ti alloys used for biomedical applications.

Alloy	R_p (MPa)	R_m (MPa)	A/Z (%)	E (GPa)
CP-Ti (grade 1–4)	170–485	240–550	15–24/25–30	−103
Ti6Al4V (annealed)	820–870	900–930	6–10/20–25	110–114
Ti6Al7Nb	880–950	900–1050	8–15/25–45	114
Ti5Al2.5Fe	895	1020	15/35	112
TAMZ	≥700	≥750	≥12%	105
Ti13Nb13Zr (aged)	830–910	970–1040	10–16/27–53	79–84
TMZF (annealed)	1000–1060	1060–1100	18–22/64–73	74–85
Ti15Mo (annealed)	544	874	21/82	78
Ti15Mo5Zr3Al (solution treated)	838	852	25/48	80
Ti35Nb5Ta7Zr	547	596	19/68	55
Ti29Nb13Ta4.6Zr	860	910	13	80
Ti2448 (aged)	800–1100	850–1150	15	42–72
TLE (solution treated)	310–365	620–760	21–39/74–83	58–73
TLE (aged)	560–1020	700–1060	15–22/67–77	58–84
TLM (solution treated)	275–500	660–705	21–26/75–84	52.6–60
TLM (aged)	610–950	685–1050	17–23/70–71	45–81
TiB12 (solution treated)	830–940	930–1040	14–20/66–77	53–80
TiB12 (aged)	960–1130	1000–1210	9–15/33–46	81–95

Source: data from Z. Yu, S. Yu, J. Cheng, X. Ma, Development and application of novel biomedical titanium alloy materials, Acta Metall Sinica 53 (2017) 1238–1264.

absorbed and metabolized by the body [33]. Degradable implant materials can be divided into degradable metals, degradable polymer materials, and degradable ceramic materials. Among them, degradable metal materials have broad application prospects in the fields of bone filling, repairing and fixation, vascular stents, tissue engineering, and so on. At present, the most studied degradable metals are magnesium-based and zinc-based materials. The typical properties of some medical metal materials are shown in Table 1.7.

1.7.1 Magnesium alloys

As a light metal, magnesium has a density close to that of human bone, and its elastic modulus is closer to that of cortical bone tissue.

1.7 Degradable metals

TABLE 1.7 Typical properties of some metal implant materials and natural bone [20,21].

Materials	ρ (g/cm^3)	E (GPa)	R_m (MPa)	R_m/ρ (MPa/g cm^{-3})	E/ρ (GPa/g cm^{-3})	R_p/R_m
Cortical bone	1.8	3–30	30–200	166	22	H
316L	8.0	193	465–950	120	25	M
TiNi	6.5	28–83	850–1250	184	12	M
CoCrMo	9.1	240–270	860–1250	137	26	M
CP–Ti	4.5	105–110	200–500	111	24	H
Ti6Al4V	4.43	114	900–1200	266	24	H
TLM	5.1	60–110	800–1200	235	22	H
Pure Mg	1.74	41–45	100–200	150	–	H
Pure Zn	7.14	75–82	200–300	250	–	H

Such property characteristics allow magnesium and its alloys to be used as biomedical materials to avoid the stress shielding effect of implant materials to the greatest extent in the repair process of bone fracture [34]. The design of medical magnesium alloys is mainly based on MgZn series; Guangyin Yuan's team at Shanghai Jiaotong University in China has developed a MgNdZnZr magnesium alloy and conducted research on the alloy in vascular stents and orthopedics [35]. Shaokang Guan's team at Zhengzhou University in China has also developed a MgZnYNd magnesium alloy and performed application research on vascular stents and other products [36]. However, as yet, none of China's domestic magnesium alloy products have been used in practical applications. Only the pure magnesium bone nails produced by Dongguan Yian Technology Co., Ltd. have been approved by the European Union's CE certification and can be sold in the European Union and related overseas markets. Dreams 2G from Biotronik of Germany was granted the EU CE certification in June 2016, becoming the first drug-eluting biodegradable magnesium alloy stent to enter the market, under the trade name Magmaris. Zhentao Yu's research group at the Northwest Institute for Nonferrous Metal Research (NIN) has conducted research on the design and processing of MgZn series magnesium alloys. Based on the Arrhenius equation and Zener–Hollomon parameters, the flow stress constitutive model of Mg3Zn1Zr alloy during high temperature deformation was established by using multiple regression analysis method [37]. With the application of Defrom-3D software, a finite element simulation analysis of the parameters of the extrusion die for a variety of Mg3Zn1Zr alloy tubes with small diameter and thin walls was carried out [38], and the effects of extrusion ratio, extrusion speed, and extrusion temperature on the formability and grain size distribution of magnesium alloy thin-walled tubes were simulated. After simulation and optimization the special extruded Mg3Zn1Zr alloy tubes with good surface quality, high dimensional accuracy, and fine and uniform grains were obtained, as shown in Fig. 1.5. It has good comprehensive mechanical properties, with a tensile strength of 280 MPa, a yield strength of 195 MPa, and elongation of 19%. In addition, studies have shown that a small amount of Zr can refine the grains of magnesium alloys, and the extruded Mg1.5Zn0.1Zr magnesium alloy has better mechanical properties, with fine and uniform grains, thus showing uniform corrosion morphology. The mouse embryonic osteoblast precursor cells (MC3T3-E1) proliferate well on it, so it has good potential for orthopedic applications.

Severe plastic deformation is an important methods for improving the performance of magnesium alloys. However, because magnesium alloys have a close-packed hexagonal crystal structure with few slip systems that can be activated at room temperature, its cold working is difficult. Zhentao Yu's research group at NIN studied the effect of hot rotary forging on the microstructure and mechanical properties of WE43 magnesium alloy [39]. After hot rotary forging, the grains and second phase structure of magnesium alloy were significantly refined, and "a processing method for small-sized magnesium alloy bars with high strength" was invented [40]. Our team studied the processing of magnesium filaments and also successfully prepared superfine magnesium wires with bright and knotted surfaces (Fig. 1.6). According to the application of degradable cerclage thread and surgical suture, "a metal ultrafine wire drawing device and a degradable metal ultrafine wire drawing method" were invented [41–43].

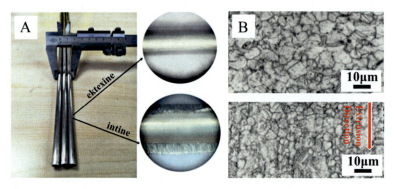

FIGURE 1.5 Mg3Zn1Zr alloy thin-diameter tubes. (A) Macro photo. (B) Microstructure.

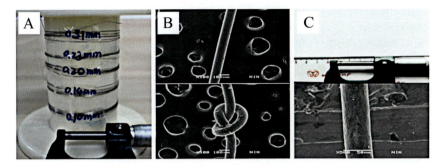

FIGURE 1.6 Mg ultrafine wire. (A) Macro view of different samples. (B) Micro view of Φ0.1 mm wire, (C) Φ50-μm wire.

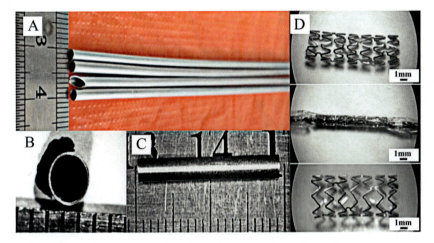

FIGURE 1.7 Zinc alloy tube (Φ2.5 × 0.13 mm) and stent with small diameters and thin walls. (A) Macro photo of tube. (B) Cross section of tube. (C) Surface photo of tube. (D) Vascular stent.

1.7.2 Zinc alloys

Zinc is the second most abundant metal element in the human body. It plays important roles in cell proliferation, the immune system, and the nervous system [44]. However, the mechanical strength of pure zinc cannot fully meet the strength requirements of the implants; therefore some alloying elements need to be added to improve its strength. Zhentao Yu's research group of NIN cooperating with Xi'an Advans Medical Technology Co., Ltd. firstly developed zinc alloy thin-walled tubes and vascular stent in China [45]. The surface of the tube is bright, the wall thickness is uniform, and the stent expands evenly without cracking (Fig. 1.7).

At present, the alloy design, research and development, and application standards of metal materials for surgical implants consider only the four basic requirements of material composition, microstructure, strength, and plasticity in addition to the requirements of qualified biosafety index. With the development of new research concepts or ideas, such as biomechanical compatibility, biological suitability, tissue suitability, mechanical suitability, and degradable suitability with body tissues, the alloy design standard requirements of medical metals and their alloy materials should also be improved accordingly. Six key aspects need to be focused on: (1) ensuring the biocompatibility of the alloy, abandoning or reducing the alloy elements that have proven toxic and side effects on the body; (2) striving to simplify the phase composition (component or structure) of the alloy and trying to avoid the formation of intermetallic compound phases; (3) improving the biomechanical compatibility of the alloy, which requires, in addition to reducing the elastic modulus of the metal material to achieve an excellent match with the lower human bone tissue, considering other comprehensive mechanical properties of the alloy, such as fatigue strength; (4) expanding the versatility and controllability of the alloy, on the one hand further developing the alloy's performance and functions such as shape memory, superelasticity, and biodegradability and on the other hand realizing the controllability of the above-mentioned functions and the match with the comprehensive properties, including strength, toughness, processing, and formability; (5) endeavoring to reduce the processing and manufacturing costs of alloys, not only to reduce the content of alloy elements with high melting and expensive price, but also to improve the easy processing and formability of the alloy; and (6) improving the quality of biomedical metal materials and launching a solid foundation for later batch applications. This requires that after the new medical metal materials have been developed and finalized, full attention should be paid to quality control in the subsequent processing and heat treatment of the alloy. Only by realizing the target requirements of biomedical metal materials, such as cleanliness, homogenization, fine crystallization, porosity, and low cost, can these materials meet the promotion and application requirements in various surgical implantation and interventional medicine fields.

References

[1] K. Yang, Y. Ren, Research and development of medical stainless steels, Materials China 12 (2010) 1–10.
[2] M. Speidel, Properties and applications of high nitrogen steels, High Nitrogen Steels—HNS 88 (1988) 92–96.
[3] Q. Wang, B. Zhang, Y. Ren, K. Yang, Research and application of biomedical nickel-free stainless steels, Acta Metallurgica Sinica 53 (2017) 1311–1316.

[4] S. Chen, M. Lü, J. Zhang, J. Dong, K. Yang, Microstructure and antibacterial properties of Cu—contained antibacterial stainless steel Cu-Al, Acta Metallurgica Sinica 40 (2004) 309—313.
[5] L. Nan, Study on antibacterial properties of copper-containing antibacterial stainless steels, Acta Metallurgica Sinica — Chinese Edition 43 (2007) 1065—1070.
[6] I.T. Hong, C.H. Koo, Antibacterial properties, corrosion resistance and mechanical properties of Cu-modified SUS 304 stainless steel, Materials Science and Engineering: A 393 (2005) 213—222.
[7] Q. Chen, G. Thouas, Metallic implant biomaterials, Materials Science and Engineering: R: Reports 87 (2015) 1—57.
[8] S. Asgari, Anomalous plastic behavior of fine-grained MP35N alloy during room temperature tensile testing, Journal of Materials Processing Technology 155 (2004) 1905—1911.
[9] C. Li, J. Oh, S. Choi, J. Hong, J. Yeom, X. Mei, et al., Study on microstructure and mechanical property of a biomedical Co-20Cr-15W-10Ni alloy during multi-pass thermomechanical processing, Materials Science and Engineering: A 785 (2020) 139388.
[10] R. Wang, R. Wang, D. Chen, G. Qin, E. Zhang, Novel CoCrWNi alloys with Cu addition: microstructure, mechanical properties, corrosion properties and biocompatibility, Journal of Alloys and Compounds 824 (2020) 153924.
[11] D. Favier, H. Louche, P. Schlosser, L. Orgéas, P. Vacher, L. Debove, Homogeneous and heterogeneous deformation mechanisms in an austenitic polycrystalline Ti—50.8 wt.% Ni thin tube under tension. Investigation *via* temperature and strain fields measurements, Acta Materialia 55 (2007) 5310—5322.
[12] H. Liu, Z. Yu, S. Yu, J. Liu, Y. Zhang, C. Wang, et al., Study on the hot compression deformation behavior of Ni—Ti shape memory alloy, Study on the hot compression deformation behavior of Ni—Ti shape memory alloy, Hot Working Technology 47 (2018) 59—63.
[13] G. Li, Research and development of precious metal materials for medical uses, Precious Metals 025 (2004) 54—61.
[14] L. Benner, Precious metals science and technology, Platinum Metals Review 35 (1991) 93.
[15] Y. Wang, Q. Cao, Z. Jia, J. Zheng, Application and development of precious metals in the field of medicine, Rare Metal Materials and Engineering 43 (2014) 165—170.
[16] W. Kean, L. Hart, W. Buchanan, Auranofin, British Journal of Rheumatology 36 (1997) 560—572.
[17] B. Rosenberg, Some biological effects of platinum compounds, Platinum Metals Review 15 (1971) 42—51.
[18] Z. Yu, S. Yu, J. Cheng, X. Ma, Development and application of novel biomedical titanium alloy materials, Acta Metallurgica Sinica 53 (2017) 1238—1264.
[19] B. Levine, S. Sporer, R. Poggie, C.J. Della Valle, J.J. Jacobs, Experimental and clinical performance of porous tantalum in orthopedic surgery, Biomaterials 27 (2006) 4671—4681.
[20] K. Sagomonyants, M. Hakim-Zargar, A. Jhaveri, M. Aronow, G. Gronowicz, Porous tantalum stimulates the proliferation and osteogenesis of osteoblasts from elderly female patients, Journal of Orthopaedic Research 29 (2011) 609—616.
[21] C. Chen, C. Zhang, X. Wang, H. Jing, Research progress in the preparation of biomedical porous tantalum, Hot Working Technology 43 (2014) 5—8.
[22] C. Luo, Experimental Study on the Effect of 3D Printing Porous Tantalum Pore Size and Porosity on Osteogenesis and Osseointegration, Chongqing Medical University, 2020.
[23] A. Tsao, J. Roberson, M. Christie, D. Dore, D. Heck, D. Robertson, et al., Biomechanical and clinical evaluations of a porous tantalum implant for the treatment of early-stage osteonecrosis, Journal of Bone & Joint Surgery 87 (2005) 22—27.

[24] T. Zhang, Y. Zhang, Q. Zhao, Application of porous tantalum metal in clinical bone and joint repair, International Journal of Orthopaedics 1 (2015) 36–39.
[25] L. Geng, H. Gan, Q. Wang, H. Zhang, Y. Liu, Z. Wang, et al., Effect of domestic porous tantalum on biocompatibility and osteogenic gene expression in rat osteoblasts, Journal of Third Military Medical University 36 (2014) 1163–1167.
[26] H. Cai, H. He, Research progress of tantalum metal in clinical application, Journal of Oral and Maxillofacial Prosthetics 18 (2017) 46–50.
[27] D. Kuroda, M. Niinomi, M. Morinaga, Y. Kato, T. Yashiro, Design and mechanical properties of new β type titanium alloys for implant materials, Materials Science and Engineering: A 243 (1998) 244–249.
[28] T. Saito, T. Furuta, J. Hwang, S. Kuramoto, K. Nishino, N. Suzuki, et al., Multifunctional alloys obtained *via* a dislocation-free plastic deformation mechanism, Science 300 (2003) 464–467.
[29] Z. Yu, L. Zhou, K. Wang, B. Zhao, Q. Hong, J. Niu, et al., A β-type titanium alloy for surgical implants, Authorization Number: ZL03153139.3 (2005).
[30] Z. Yu, L. Zhou, K. Wang, Q. Hong, B. Zhao, J. Niu, et al., A β-type titanium alloy for vascular stent, Authorization Number: ZL03153138.5 (2005).
[31] J. Niu, Z. Yu, S. Liu, X. He, Y. Zhang, J. Han, et al., A metastable β titanium alloy with low elastic modulus, Authorization Number: ZL201110184053.X (2012).
[32] Y. Hao, R. Yang, High strength nano-structure Ti-Nb-Sn alloy, Acta Metallurgica Sinica 41 (2005) 1183–1189.
[33] R. Narayan, Biomedical Materials, Springer Science & Business Media, 2009.
[34] Y. Chen, Z. Xu, C. Smith, J. Sankar, Recent advances on the development of magnesium alloys for biodegradable implants, Acta Biomaterialia 10 (2014) 4561–4573.
[35] H. Qin, Y. Zhao, Z. An, M. Cheng, Q. Wang, T. Cheng, et al., Enhanced antibacterial properties, biocompatibility, and corrosion resistance of degradable Mg-Nd-Zn-Zr alloy, Biomaterials 53 (2015) 211–220.
[36] J. Wang, L. Wang, S. Guan, S. Zhu, C. Ren, S. Hou, Microstructure and corrosion properties of as sub-rapid solidification Mg–Zn–Y–Nd alloy in dynamic simulated body fluid for vascular stent application, Journal of Materials Science: Materials in Medicine 21 (2010) 2001–2008.
[37] C. Wang, Z. Yu, Z. Yu, X. Zhao, P. Xu, X. Dai, Hot deformation behavior and constitutive model of Mg-3Zn-1Zr alloy, Light Metal 12 (2018) 43–47.
[38] C. Wang, Z. Yu, Z. Yu, B.W. Zhao X., Y. Wang, Extrusion die design of Mg-3Zn-Zr alloy thin tube, Materials Reports 32 (2018) 350–354.
[39] C. Wang, Z. Yu, Y. Cui, S. Yu, H. Liu, Effect of hot rotary swaging and subsequent annealing on microstructure and mechanical properties of magnesium alloy WE43, Metal Science and Heat Treatment 60 (2019) 777–782.
[40] C. Wang, Z. Yu, Y. Wang, H. Liu, Y. Zhang, W. Lan, A high-strength magnesium alloy small-size bar processing method, Authorization Number: ZL201611037633.5 (2017).
[41] C. Wang, D. Ai, Z. Yu, S. Liu, Finite element simulation of pure magnesium wire drawing, Special Casting and Nonferrous Alloys 38 (2005) 850–852.
[42] C. Wang, D. Ai, Z. Yu, S. Luo, X. Dai, H. Liu, et al., Research on the cold drawing process of pure magnesium filaments, Light Metal 7 (2019) 40–43.
[43] C. Wang, Z. Yu, J. Niu, B. Wen, S. Liu, W. He, et al., A metal ultrafine wire drawing device and a degradable metal ultrafine wire drawing method. Application number: CN201810274306.4, 2018.
[44] H. Tapiero, K. Tew, Trace elements in human physiology and pathology: zinc and metallothioneins, Biomedicine & Pharmacotherapy 57 (2003) 399–411.
[45] C. Wang, Z. Yu, Y. Cui, Y. Zhang, S. Yu, G. Qu, et al., Processing of a novel Zn alloy micro-tube for biodegradable vascular stent application, Journal of Materials Science & Technology 32 (2016) 925–929.

CHAPTER 2

Design and physical metallurgy of biomedical β-Ti alloys

2.1 Overview of design methods of biomedical Ti alloys

The alloy design in advance is essential for the development of high-performance biomedical β-Ti alloys. According to their microstructure and characteristics, Ti alloys can be classified into three main categories: α-type alloys, β-type alloys, and α + β-type alloys. For surgical implants, the α-type alloys [e.g., commercial pure Ti (CP-Ti) and Ti3Al2.5V] and α + β alloys (e.g., Ti6Al4V, Ti6Al7Nb, and Ti5Al2.5Fe) have been studied, developed, and applied successfully. However, these Ti alloys generally contain elements that have toxic effects on living organisms (e.g., V, Al, and Fe), and their elastic modulus is still much larger than that of natural bones (1–30 GPa), which can lead to stress shielding. This results in osteolysis and resorption around implants and loosening or fracture of the implants, finally leading to their premature failure. Therefore the United States, Japan, and China have taken the lead in research and development of new β biomedical Ti alloys with excellent biocompatibility, smaller elastic modulus, and better overall performance to meet the clinical requirements for the development and application of surgical implanting and interventional products [1].

For the new type of Ti alloys for surgical implants, the relationships between chemical composition, microstructure, and mechanical properties of β-Ti alloys are complicated because β-Ti alloys involve the interaction of many alloying elements and exhibit complex structure and physical and chemical properties. For the design theory of biomedical β-Ti alloys with high strength and low modulus, the biological and mechanical compatibility is the key indicator of the surgical Ti-based implants. Metallurgical properties, processing properties, and cost of processing and manufacturing should be also considered to meet the practical application requirements of different surgical implant products [2].

2.1.1 d-Electron theory for Ti alloy design

In the design of biomedical Ti alloys, the d-electron alloy design method is based on the positions of different types of Ti alloys in the electron orbital phase diagram and on the arrangement of elastic modulus and strength in the phase diagram. The general design criterion is first to determine the ranges or values of the electron orbital parameters of the alloy with low modulus. Then, according to the electron orbital parameters of different alloying elements and the d-electron theory, the average electron orbital parameters of the alloy are calculated to meet the design goal as shown in Fig. 2.1.

Fig. 2.1 shows the phase diagram of binary Ti alloy corresponding to electron orbital parameters of the alloying elements. The d-electron alloy design method is also called new phase analysis algorithm (NEW PHACOMP, or phase computation), which was developed on the basis of DV-Xa cluster molecular orbital calculation. In this theory, two parameters, the bond order (*Bo*) and the metal d-orbital energy level (*Md*), are used to control the phase stability and performance of alloys. *Bo* is used to characterize the strength of the covalent bonds between Ti and the alloying elements, and *Md* is a parameter related to the electronegativity of the elements and radius of the metallic bonds. The *Bo* and *Md* values of different alloying elements in β-Ti alloys are listed in Table 2.1.

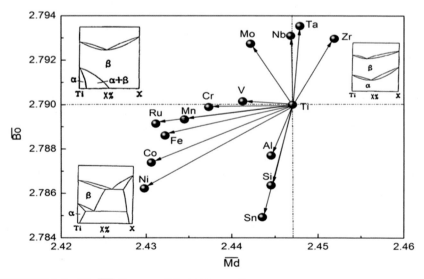

FIGURE 2.1 $\overline{Bo}-\overline{Md}$ diagram of Ti–M binary alloys.

TABLE 2.1 Bo and Md values of BCC-Ti.

	Element	Bo	Md (eV)
3d	Ti	2.790	2.447
	V	2.805	1.872
	Cr	2.779	1.478
	Mn	2.723	1.194
	Fe	2.651	0.960
	Co	2.529	0.807
	Ni	2.412	0.724
	Cu	2.112	0.567
4d	Zr	3.086	2.934
	Nb	3.099	2.424
	Mo	3.063	1.961
5d	Hf	3.110	2.975
	Ta	3.144	2.531
	W	3.125	2.072
	Al	2.426	2.200
	Si	2.561	2.200
	Sn	2.283	2.100

According to the d-electron theory, the average values of Bo and Md of alloys are defined as in Eqs. (2.1) and (2.2), respectively [3]:

$$\overline{Bo} = \sum_{i=1}^{n} x_i (Bo)_i \qquad (2.1)$$

$$\overline{Md} = \sum_{i=1}^{n} x_i (Md)_i \qquad (2.2)$$

where x_i, $(Bo)_i$, and $(Md)_i$ are the atomic fraction of alloying element i, the $\overline{Bo}$ value, and the $\overline{Md}$ value, respectively. These and their corresponded alloy and elastic modulus of some typical elements of Ti alloy are shown in Fig. 2.2. The α, $\alpha + \beta$, and β alloys are clearly divided into three regions. In the region of the β alloy, the elastic modulus of the alloy decreases with increasing $\overline{Bo}$ and $\overline{Md}$ values. Thus the high values of $\overline{Bo}$ and $\overline{Md}$ should be chosen for the design and development of new

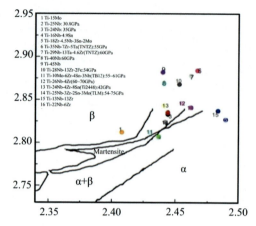

FIGURE 2.2 The position of common medical low-E Ti alloys in the phase stability diagram.

TABLE 2.2 Bo, Md, [Mo]$_{Eq}$, and E of several common biomedical Ti alloys.

Alloy designation	$\overline{Bo}$	$\overline{Md}$	[Mo]$_{Eq}$	E
Ti13Nb13Zr	2.837	2.483	3.6	79
Ti25Nb3Zr2Sn3Mo (TLM)	2.843	2.441	9.9	54
Ti29Nb13Ta4.6Zr (TNTZ)	2.878	2.462	10.98	50
Ti24Nb4Zr8Sn (Ti2448)	2.824	2.442	6.72	42
Ti12Mo6Zr2Fe (TMZF)	2.816	2.404	12	80

types of β-Ti alloys with high strength and low modulus. For Ti–M (M represents the alloying element) binary alloys, the position of the alloys in the diagram varies with the change of alloying element content. The electron orbit parameters, Mo equivalent, and elastic modulus of several common biomedical β-Ti alloys are given in Table 2.2.

At present, the d-electron alloy design theory is one of the common methods for Ti alloy design and evaluation [4]. Some new biomedical β-Ti alloys with low modulus have been designed successfully according to this method. It has been proved that the lower *Md* value is beneficial to the phase stability and the higher Bo value is good for the enhancement effect of solid solution. During the plastic processing, the main deformation mode of the thermally stable Ti alloys is slip deformation, whereas the metastable β-Ti alloys can be come into being *via* slip, twinning, and martensite deformation during plastic processing. The material mechanical properties can be adjusted in a wide range by controlling different process and microstructure of the alloys. In consequence, for the design of metastable β-Ti alloys, the *Md* and *Bo* values should be kept in the ranges 2.35–2.45 and 2.75–2.85, respectively, which requires strict control of the alloying elements, especially β-stabilizing elements and their contents [1,2]. This is because that the excessive addition of the β-stabilizing elements such as Pd, Ta, Hf, and Mo increases the alloy cost and specific gravity, easily results in melting segregations and inclusions, and is also not conducive to the formation of metastable β-Ti alloys, owing to the increased stabilization of the β phases.

2.1.2 Mo equivalent for Ti alloy design

At present, Mo equivalent calculations are often used in the design of Ti alloys. The empirical formula used to calculate the Mo equivalent is slightly different between China, Russia, and the United States. The commonly used Mo equivalent calculation formulas are as follows:

$$[Mo]_{eq} = \%[Mo] + \%[V]/1.5 + \%[W]/2 \\ + \%[Nb]/3.6 + \%[Ta]/4.5 \\ + \%[Fe]/0.35 + \%[Cr]/0.63 \\ + \%[Mn]/0.65 + \%[Ni]/0.8 \\ - \%[Al] \text{(The United States)} \quad (2.3)$$

$$[Mo]_{eq} = \%[Mo] + \%[V]/1.4 + \%[W]/2 \\ + \%[Nb]/3.3 + \%[Ta]/4 + \%[Fe]/0.5 \\ + \%[Cr]/0.6 + \%[Mn]/0.6 + \%[Ni]/0.8 \\ + \%[Co]/0.9 \text{(Russia)} \quad (2.4)$$

$$[Mo]_{eq} = 1.0Mo + 0.67V + 0.44W + 0.28Nb \\ + 0.22Ta + 1.6Cr + \cdots - 1.0Al \text{(China)} \quad (2.5)$$

By calculating the Mo equivalent of the β-Ti alloys to be designed, the influence of various alloying elements on the phase stability can be obtained preliminarily, and then the microstructure and mechanical properties of β-Ti alloys can be predicted. The common β-stabilizing elements and related design parameters are shown in Table 2.3. Therefore the Mo equivalent design is a practical and efficient alloy design method for the development of new types of β-Ti alloys. According to the calculated Mo equivalent value, content of the added β-stabilizing elements, and microstructure characteristics, the designed biomedical β-Ti alloys can be subdivided into three categories: near β-type, metastable β-type, and stable β-type. It has been found that [1,2] when the Mo equivalent value of the alloy is between 2.8 (e.g., Ti10Nd35Zr) and 23 (e.g., Ti13V11Cr3Al), the designed alloy generally belongs to the

TABLE 2.3 Influence of critical concentration β_c of commonly used stabilization elements on phase transition temperature T_β of Ti alloys.

β-stabilizer	Mo	V	W	Nb	Ta	Fe	Cr	Ni	Mn	Co
β_c (wt.%)	10.0	15	22.5	36	45	3.5	6.3	9	6.4	7
T_β (°C/wt.%)	−8.3	−5.5	−13.8	−10.6	−15.6	18	15	22	22	21

metastable or near β-Ti alloys. When the Mo equivalent is smaller than 2.8, the alloy tends to form α + β two-phase Ti alloys. When the Mo equivalent is larger than 30, a stable complete β-type Ti alloys will be formed. Metastable β-Ti alloys and near β-Ti alloys belong to mesostable β-Ti alloys, which generally have the characteristics of high specific strength matching with high toughness, low modulus, better properties in hardenability, corrosion resistance, cold formability, and heat treatment hardening. Compared to the α-Ti and α + β-Ti alloys, the density of the mesostable β-Ti alloys increase slightly, but the strength, toughness, corrosion resistance, and cold and hot formability are higher or better than those of the α + β-Ti alloys, while the elastic modulus and fatigue notch sensitivity are lower than those of the α-Ti and α + β-Ti alloys.

2.2 Overview of composition design of biomedical Ti alloys

There appears to be a series of biological effects after metal elements enter the human body. According to their different effects on the human body, metal elements can be divided into three categories: essential elements, harmful elements, and toxic elements. Even for essential elements, their concentration in the human body has a maximum limit. Once the concentration is beyond its maximum limit, essential elements will also become harmful elements. Table 2.4 summarizes the biological effects and characteristics of common metal elements in the human body [5]. For the human body, essential elements can maintain the dynamic balance in the body by regulating one or more metabolic processes. Harmful elements and toxic elements can simply accumulate and be slowly metabolized in certain tissues and organs instead of exhibiting the regulatory effect. In addition, there is obvious selectivity for the distribution of chemical elements in various tissues of the human body, so the specific application of Ti alloys in different parts of the human body should be considered in the alloy design.

From the point of view of the β-stabilizing elements, an appropriate number of β-stabilizing elements should be added to the alloy to retain

TABLE 2.4 Biological effects and characteristics of common metal elements in the human body.

Element	Feature	Content (mg)	Function	Excessive reaction
Fe	Necessary	4×10^3	Promotes metabolism and compose proteins	Iron poisoning, liver and kidney damage
Mo	Necessary	9	Promotes metabolism and compose enzymes	Molybdenum poisoning, bone abnormalities
Cu	Necessary	100	Promotes metabolism and compose enzymes	Copper poisoning, hemolysis
Al	Harmful	100	Interferes with metabolism and bone lesions	Interferes with phosphorus absorption and affects nerves
V	Necessary	3×10^{-5}	Participates in oxidation-reduction reactions	Vanadium poisoning, liver and kidney damage
Co	Necessary	1.1	Participates in enzyme activities	Affects heart function
Ni	Necessary	10	Increases insulin and lowers blood sugar	Damage to respiratory tract, nose cancer
Cr	Necessary	6		Chromium poisoning, cancer

the β phase at room temperature after quenching. The stabilizing elements that can be added in Ti alloys include isomorphism elements Mo, V, Nb, Ta, and so on and eutectoid elements Cu, Mn, Cr, Fe, Ni, Co, and so on. In addition, the neutral elements Sn and Zr are also commonly added to β-Ti alloys. From the perspective of cytotoxicity, Al, V, Cu, Ni, Co, Cr, and so on have potential toxicity, while Nb, Ta, Zr, Sn, Pd, Hf, and so on have good biocompatibility, as concluded from studies on the cytotoxicity of pure metals and the relationship between the biocompatibility of pure metals and surgical implant alloys and their polarization resistance [3].

Generally speaking, the α-stabilizing elements, such as Al, O, and N, are very effective in strengthening Ti alloys, but they usually reduce the toughness and increase the elastic modulus of materials. However, Zr, Nb, Mo, and Sn can strengthen the Ti matrix, have less adverse effect on the toughness, and at the same time benefit the reduction in elastic modulus. To meet the design requirements of the composition diversification and biomechanical performance matching of new types of β-Ti alloys, special attention should be paid to the coupling effect of alloy diversification on properties. Furthermore, the alloying elements, especially the β-stabilizing elements and their ratio (weight or atomic ratio), should be strictly selected and controlled. It has been confirmed that the effects of Zr, Sn, Mo, Nb, and Ta elements on the physical and chemical properties, such as strength, plasticity, and modulus, of multicomponent Ti alloys have a nonlinear or quantitative relationship with the ratio of the elements in the alloys. Different elements have different effects on the properties of the alloys, and the variations in mechanical properties become more complex with the change in the alloy composition, which is different from the influences of binary alloys [1]. Gaseous impurity elements such as O and N increase the elastic modulus while improving the strength of the alloy. Therefore they are usually added as trace elements to adjust the plasticity, toughness, and elastic modulus. Although the Hf, Ta, and Nb elements have good biological safety and are beneficial to the low modulus and regulation of plasticity and toughness of alloys, these materials have a high melting point and are expensive.

Generally speaking, for Ti alloys, with increases in its strength, modulus, hardness, wear resistance, and fatigue properties, its plasticity, toughness (fracture and impact), and machinability decline. These multiple contradictions make the comprehensive matching of biomechanical properties of biomedical Ti alloys more complex. The secondary optimal design of multicomponent alloys must be carried out by taking into account the aspects of alloy melting, cold and hot processing, heat treatment, and control of microstructure and mechanical properties of biomedical Ti alloys.

In addition to biocompatibility and the effects of alloying elements on microstructure and mechanical properties, the low cost and wider processing window of the new types of β-Ti alloys with high strength and low modulus should also be taken into account. For example, Hf, Ta, and Nb elements should be added with caution. The addition of the Fe element should be minimized because Fe will hinder radiation and is not conducive to the postoperative CT or MRI examination of patients. At present, nearly 100 new types of biomedical Ti alloys have been reported at home and abroad, and the novel alloy developing includes binary to six-component alloys with nearly 20 alloying elements involved. The designs of common components of biomedical Ti alloys are summarized in Table 2.5 [6].

2.3 Overview of the design and development of typical biomedical β-Ti alloys

In the past 20 years, given their excellent biocompatibility, high specific strength, high processing plasticity, and elastic modulus similar to

2.3 Overview of the design and development of typical biomedical β-Ti alloys

TABLE 2.5 Composition design of various biomedical β-Ti alloys.

Alloy series	Alloy components
Binary alloy	TiMo, TiNb, TiTa, TiHf, TiZr
Ternary alloys	TiNbPt, TiNbPd, TiNbTa, TiNbZr, TiNbHf, TiNbFe, TiNbSn, TiNbO, TiNbAl; TiMoTa, TiMoNb, TiMoSn, TiMoHf, TiMoGa, TiMoAl, TiMoGe, TiMoAg, TiTaFe, TiTaZr
Quaternary alloys	TiNbTaZr, TiNbTaSn, TiNbMoZr, TiMoZrSn, TiMoZrFe, TiMoZrAl, TiMoNbSn, TiMoGaNb, TiTaZrFe, TiMoNbSi, TiMoNbO
Quinary alloys	TiMoNbZrSn, TiMoAlNbSi, TiNbSnTaPd, TiNbZrTaO
Quaternary alloys	Ti12Ta9Nb3V6Zr1.5O, Ti23Nb0.7Ta2Zr1.2O, TiFeMoMnNbZr

that of human bone tissue, the novel biomedical low-modulus β-Ti alloys have been continuously studied worldwide, and the feasibility of their applications for human hard tissue repair and replacement have been actively explored. Researchers in the United States, Japan, China, and some other countries have developed more than 20 new low-modulus β-Ti alloys, including TiNb-based, TiMo-based, TiZr-based, and TiTa-based multicomponent alloys. Among them, those that have been included in international standards are Ti13Nb13Zr (ASTM F 1713), Ti12Mo6Zr2Fe (ASTM F 1813), Ti15Mo (ASTM F 2066), Ti15Mo5Zr3Al (JIS T 7401-6), Ti45Nb (AMS 4982), Ti2.5Al5Mo5V (VT 16), Ti5Al2Sn (VT 5-1), Ti35Nb7Zr5Ta (Task force F-04.12.23), and Ti30Ta [1].

The Northwest Institute for Nonferrous Metal Research (NIN) of China has been committed to the design and development of various biomedical Ti alloys since 1980s and is at the forefront of international industrial applications of Ti alloys. The novel biomedical Ti alloys, including Ti2.5Al2.5Mo2.5Zr (TAMZ), Ti3Zr2Sn3Mo25Nb (TLM), Ti15Nb5Zr3Mo (TLE), and Ti10Mo6Zr4Sn3Nb (TB12), have been developed and obtained Chinese national invention patents since 1999. In 2002 the research and development group lead by Professor Zhentao Yu developed two new types of metastable β-Ti alloys, TLM (Ti alloy with low modulus) and TLE (Ti alloy with low E), supported by the National High Technology Research and Development Program (863 Program of China). Their design principles were as follows: (1) The alloying elements with lower cost that are nontoxic, fully solid solubilized in α-Ti and β-Ti matrix, and the TiNb binary system were selected as the basic system of alloy design. (2) Using the methods of combining the d-electron theory and Mo equivalent empirical formula, the design parameters that can appear as a metastable phase transition and martensite transformation and the mesostable phase of alloy at room temperature were reserved according to the phase diagrams of binary phase and d-electron orbit of Ti alloys. (3) Based on the first principles, the effects of the Sn, Zr, and Mo alloying elements and their contents on the strength, modulus, and martensitic transformation temperature were calculated. Giving full consideration to the cold and hot processing and forming characteristics of Ti alloys in advance, these novel biomedical β-Ti alloys with high strength and low modulus were obtained through a series of industrial experiments [2], and their comprehensive mechanical properties can be adjusted in a wide range according to the practical application. Some new β-type Ti alloys that have been designed and developed in China for biomedical applications are listed in Table 2.6.

TABLE 2.6 Some typical β-T alloys designed and developed in China.

Alloys	Alloy type	Alloy design and typical features	Remarks
Ti24Nb4Zr7.9Sn (Ti2448)	Near β	Electron concentration 4.15; medium strength, low modulus of elasticity and Poisson's ratio	Used in orthopedic devices by Chinese Academy of Sciences Institute of Metal
Ti3Zr2Sn3Mo25Nb (TLM)	Near β	d-Electron theory and Mo equivalent design, medium and high strength, low modulus, easy machining	Used in orthopedic, dental, and vascular stents by NIN
Ti5Zr3Mo25Nb (TLE)	Near β	High strength, low modulus, easy to process	Used in orthopedic, dental, and vascular stents by NIN
Ti10Mo6Zr4Sn3Nb (TB12)	Near β	High strength, low modulus, easy to process	Used in orthopedic, dental devices by NIN
Ti26Nb20Ta	Metastable β	d-Electron theory, low modulus, high workability	Beijing University of Technology
Ti22Nb4Zr2Sn	Near β	d-Electron theory, low modulus, memory effect and hyperelasticity, good cold deformation	Tianjin University
Ti11Nb (11−21) Zr Ti (15−30) Mo7Zr	Metastable β	Cluster line matching method, low modulus	Dalian University of Technology
Ti34Nb6ZrTi28Nb25Zr	Near β	d-Electron theory, low modulus, corrosion resistance	Tianjin University
Ti35Nb10Zr Ti35Nb8Zr2Mo	Metastable β	d-Electron theory, low modulus, corrosion resistance	
Ti20Nb15Zr10Mo	Metastable β	Low modulus	Hebei University of Technology
Ti39Nb5Ta7Zr	Metastable β	d-Electron theory, low modulus	Harbin Institute of Technology
Ti7.5Nb1Sn (1−6) Mo	Near β	d-Electron theory, Mo equivalent, low modulus, memory effects and hyperelasticity	Xiangtan University

Ti13Nb13Zr, Ti12Mo6Zr2Fe (TMZF), and Ti15Mo were first designed and developed in the United States to reduce the stress shielding effect and improve biomechanical compatibility [7]. Ti15Mo5Zr3Al was designed by Kobe Steel, Ltd. based on Ti15Mo in accordance with the requirements of improving strength and corrosion resistance. Ti45Nb alloy was originally designed in the United States according to the requirements of aerospace components, such as fasteners, and subsequently was introduced into the field of biomedical engineering because of its high strength, low modulus, and good corrosion resistance. With the continuous applications of low-modulus Ti alloys, Japan has carried out much research and development work. The metastable β-Ti alloy Ti29Nb13Ta4.6Zr (TNTZ) with a minimum elastic modulus of about 55 GPa was developed by Datong Steel Co. Ltd. based on the DV-Xα theory and d-electron alloy design method. To reduce the cost and elastic modulus of TNTZ alloy and improve its strength and fatigue performance, Professor Niinomi's research group [8–10] also optimized the comprehensive mechanical properties of the alloy, such as strength, elastic modulus, plasticity, and superelasticity, by adding the O and Cr elements with different contents and by adopting methods such as large plastic deformation, cumulative continuous cold rolling, deformation-induced phase transition, and thermal mechanical treatment. They revealed the reduction of modulus of TNTZ alloy with increasing high-pressure torsion or texture and the dependence of single-crystal TNTZ on crystal orientation. The elastic modulus of the TNTZ alloy increases from 64 to 77 GPa by increasing the O content to suppress the generation of heat-free ω phase and by increasing the Cr element and alloy cold deformation. Therefore they put forward the design method of Ti alloys with the self-regulating modulus for spine fixation devices and developed a series of alloys, including TiCr, Ti17Mo, Ti30Zr5Cr, Ti30Zr7Mo, and Ti30Zr3Mo3Cr. Most of the low-modulus Ti alloys designed by Japanese researchers have been developed on the basis of TNTZ and were designed and studied mainly by changing the alloying elements and their components and based on the low-cost concept, and their applications are not limited to the field of biomedical engineering. Table 2.7 lists the major types of Ti alloys developed at home and abroad and their typical mechanical properties.

In recent years, applications of Ti alloys in the biomedical field have been developing rapidly, which requires higher performance for Ti alloys. The future design and development directions of novel biomedical Ti alloys can be summarized as follows [11–14]: (1) the development of biomedical Ti alloys with monocrystalline grown in a certain direction to obtain an elastic modulus very close to that of human bone and better strength and modulus matching when used in implants; (2) the adjusting and controlling of microstructure and properties of Ti alloys

TABLE 2.7 The typical β-Ti alloys and their mechanical properties developed worldwide.

Country	Alloys	Alloy types	Typical performance
United States	Ti13Nb13Zr	Near β	R_m = 1030 MPa, A = 15%, E = 79 GPa
	Ti12Mo6Zr2Fe (TMZF)	Metastable β	R_m = 1000 MPa, A = 10%, E = 74–85 GPa
	Ti35Nb5Ta7Zr	Near β	R_m = 599 MPa, A = 19%, E = 55 GPa
	Ti35Nb5Ta7Zr0.40	Near β	R_m = 1010 MPa, E = 66 GPa
	Ti15Mo3Nb0.3OSi	Metastable β	R_m = 1034 MPa, A = 14%, E = 79–83 GPa
	Ti15Mo3Nb3Al	Metastable β	R_m = 812 MPa, E = 82 GPa
	Ti16Nb10Hf (Tiadyne1610)	Near β	R_m = 851 MPa, A = 10%, E = 81 GPa
	Ti35Zr10Nb	Near β	R_m = 1050 MPa, A = 14%, E = 80 GPa
	Ti15Mo	Metastable	R_m = 874 MPa, A = 21%, E = 78 GPa
Japan	Ti15Mo5Zr3Al	Metastable β	R_m = 975 MPa, A = 25%, E = 75 GPa
	Ti29Nb13Ta4.6Zr (TNTZ)	Metastable β	R_m = 911 MPa, A = 13%, E = 65 GPa
	Ti12Ta9Nb3V6Zr1.5O Ti23Nb0.7Ta2Zr1.2O (Gum metal)	Near β	R_m ≤ 2100 MPa, A = 20–60 GPa, ε_c ≤ 99.9%
	Ti15Zr (Sn)4Nb2Ta0.2Pa	Near β	R_m = 726–990 MPa, A = 14–24, E = 94–99 GPa
	Ti15Zr4Nb4Ta	Near β	R_m = 1000 MPa, A = 10%, Z50%
	Ti25Nb11Sn	Near β	R_p = 1000 MPa, A = 20–40 GPa
China	Ti3ZrMo15Nb (TLE)	Near β	R_m = 900 MPa, R = 795 MPa, $A\%$ = 18%, E = 71 GPa
	Ti3Zr2Sn3Mo25Nb (TLM)	Near β	R_m = 600–1000 MPa, $A\%$ = 22%–39%, E = 54–78 GPa
	Ti11Mo5Zr4Sn3Nb (TB12)	Metastable β	R_m = 970–1020 MPa, $A\%$ = 18%, E = 56 GPa
	Ti24Nb4Zr8Sn (Ti2448)	Metastable β	R_m = 850 MPa, $A\%$ = 18%, E = 42 GPa
	Ti17Nb16Zr1Fe	Metastable β	R_m ≥ 650 MPa, $A\%$ ≥ 15%, E ≤ 65 GPa

with multiple functions such as superelasticity or shape memory effect; (3) the study of biomechanical compatibility of finer-grain Ti alloys with high strength and low modulus and their applications; (4) improvement of the mechanical properties of biomedical porous Ti alloys while reducing their modulus by regulating the porosity; (5) research and development of novel bio-Ti alloys with multiple functions (antibacterial, superelastic, shape memory, etc.) and low cost.

2.4 Smelting and physical metallurgical properties of typical β-Ti alloys

2.4.1 Review of the smelting of β-type Ti alloys

Because of their high chemical activity, Ti and its alloys in the high-temperature molten state can react with many metals and inorganic materials, resulting in material pollution. Therefore the melting of Ti and its alloys must be carried out under the protection of vacuum or inert gas. The melting technologies of Ti alloys mainly include vacuum self-consuming melting and vacuum nonconsumed melting. The equipment of vacuum self-consuming melting mainly includes vacuum arc remelting (VAR), electroslag remelting (ESR), and vacuum skull furnace. The equipment of vacuum nonconsumed arc melting mainly includes vacuum nonconsumed arc remelting (VNAR), electron beam melting (EBM), plasma beam melting (PBM), and vacuum induction melting (VIM). VAR technology is the most commonly used melting method for industrial Ti alloys. EBM and PBM melting methods can also be used in the aerospace and military fields for special purposes that require high cleanliness and low inclusions. At present, the industrial production of biomedical Ti and its alloys mainly adopts a preparation method combining VAR and VIM remelting in China.

Biomedical β-Ti alloys commonly incorporate high-density, high melting−point metals such as Mo, Ta, and Nb. Therefore it is important to ensure that the alloy ingots are free of segregation and inclusions and have high cleanliness during the melting process. Generally speaking, the alloying elements of Mo, Ta, and Nb should be added as master alloys. This means that the NbTi, TiMo, and TiTa master alloys are first prepared and are then mixed with Ti sponge in the form of alloy packages, and pressed to form the consumable electrodes. Finally, the consumable electrodes are smelted in a vacuum arc furnace twice to three times to obtain Ti alloy ingots with uniform composition. For the melting of the β-Ti alloys, the melting current should be appropriately increased, the feeding time should be extended, and the high vacuum should be maintained compared to the conventional Ti alloys. Table 2.8 shows the process characteristics and parameter comparison of the common melting techniques of Ti alloys [15].

After the biomedical Ti alloy design has been finalized, the theoretical and technical foundation can be laid to achieve the desired microstructure and performance *via* the subsequent processing and heat treatment if the metallurgical quality of the Ti alloy materials is first guaranteed. As a result, it is necessary to understand the melting process, solidification

TABLE 2.8 Comparison of several vacuum melting methods for Ti alloys.

	EBM	PBM	VAR	VNAR	ESR
Material status	Slice, bar	Slice, bar	Bulk	Slice	Slice, bar
Ingot size	All sizes	All size	All size	Small size	All sizes
Deaeration effect	Optimum	Limited	Limited	Limited	Limited
Vacuum (Pa)	0.133–0.1	Inert gas	0.013–6.65	Inert gas	Inert gas
Composition control	Better	Better	Good	Better	Good
Surface quality	Good	Good	General	General	Better
Melting rate (kg h^{-1})	500–1800	600–900	800–2000	300–800	/
Foundry returns using	Larger	Larger	Limited	Larger	Limited
Specific energy consume	Larger	Larger	Smaller	Larger	Bigger
Manipulation difficulty	Hard	Hard	Easy	Easy	Hard
Equipment investment	Highest	Higher	Low	Low	Low

EBM, Electron beam melting; *ESR*, electroslag remelting; *PBM*, plasma beam melting; *VAR*, vacuum arc remelting; *VNAR*, vacuum nonconsumed arc remelting.

behavior, and formation mechanisms of metallurgical defects of Ti alloys as well as the effects of the alloy composition (main and auxiliary elements and gas impurities), their content ratio, and their microstructure (phase transformation, metallurgical defects, etc.)

The solidification structure of alloys in the VAR process is determined mainly by the alloy composition and cooling conditions. After the alloy composition has been determined, the alloy solidification structure is controlled mainly by the heat transfer conditions. The solidification structure of Ti alloy ingots prepared by VAR generally includes three crystal regions: the fine crystal region on the surface, the columnar crystal region in the subsurface layer or intermediate layer of the ingot, and the equiaxed crystal region in the center of the ingot. The morphology of grains in different crystal regions will affect the final performance of the ingot [16]. Solute redistribution is prone to occur during alloy solidification, and chemical composition segregation is an inevitable result of solute redistribution. The macrosegregation is manifested mainly in the composition difference between the inside and outside of the ingot or between the upper and lower parts. The long-range convection of the liquid phase has an important influence on the macrosegregation in the alloy. Studies on the segregation behavior of β-Ti alloy ingots with high Mo content found that crystal segregation can be prevented and controlled by regulating of Ti ingot dimensions and specification, selecting the types of master alloys and precisely controlling the melting times and current [17], and thus the Ti alloy ingots with high composition uniformity, without macrosegregation and microsegregation, which lays the foundation for the subsequent cold or hot pressure processing.

The formation of metallurgical defects in the melting process of Ti alloys is inseparable from the macrosegregation such as white spots and tree ring segregation in the ingot structure. Macrosegregation is reflected in the composition difference between the inside and outside of the ingot or between the upper and lower parts. There are always some macroshrinkage or microshrinkage pores in the head, middle, grain boundary, and interdendritic regions of the ingot smelted by VAR. The shrinkage pores that are large and concentrated are called shrinkage cavities, while those that are small and scattered are called shrinkage porosity, and the shrinkage porosity that occurs at the grain boundary or between dendrites is called microshrinkage porosity. There is stress concentration at any shrinkage porosity or shrinkage cavity, which will not only significantly reduce the mechanical properties of the ingot, but also lead to cracks during the ingot cogging process. Microshrinkage porosity can generally be compounded in the subsequent deep processing, whereas the shrinkage cavity with gas and nonmetallic inclusions cannot generally be bonded and only elongated and even more will cause the processing crack or delamination of the ingot along the shrinkage cavity. These defects, such as peeling and bubbles formed during subsequent annealing process, will reduce the surface quality and yield of the product [18].

The numerical simulation of the ingot melting process is the intersection of materials, physics, mathematics, and computer graphics, which is also at the forefront of advanced manufacturing technology. The numerical simulation of the ingot melting process can help engineers and technicians optimize process parameters, shorten the experiment period, reduce production costs, and ensure the quality of ingots. The Pro CAST software can be used to numerically simulate the shrinkage porosity and cavity of the ingot after solidification and to initially determine the actual location of the shrinkage porosity and cavity in the ingot [19–21]. At present, the numerical calculation of the VAR process has entered the stage of multiphysics and multiscale coupling at home and abroad, and it is useful for revealing the scientific rules on melt flow, heat transfer, electromagnetic effect, microstructure, and formation of melting defects during VAR process and thus guiding the quality control of metallurgy of Ti alloy ingots.

2.4.2 TiTa alloys

Scholars from domestic and foreign regions have carried out extensive research on the design and development of TixTa alloy. Fedotov et al. systematically studied the relationship between the phase transformation during high-temperature quenching and composition of TiTa binary alloys [22]. When the tantalum content is increased, the α, α″, ω, and β phases are formed sequentially, and the β phase gradually increases. When the content of Ta exceeds 65 wt.%, all the phases will transform into the β phase. Zhou et al. studied the microstructure and mechanical properties of TiTa binary alloys and found that the quenched Ti30Ta and Ti70Ta alloys have lower Young's modulus of 69 and 67 GPa, respectively, and the corresponding tensile strength is 587 and 600 MPa, respectively [23]. It can be concluded that increasing the content of the expensive and high melting–point Ta element cannot significantly reduce the elastic modulus of the alloy, and the tensile strength is also at a lower level. Margevicius et al. found that the yield platform of the Ti60Ta alloy during the tensile test is caused by the stress-induced martensitic transformation [24]. During the high-temperature quenching process, the ω phase is precipitated, the volume fraction of the ω precipitation phase goes up with increasing the heat treatment temperature, and the precipitation of the ω phase will hinder the β→α″ martensitic transformation. Studies on the corrosion resistance of Ta alloys have revealed that the stability of Ta_2O_5 was better than that of TiO_2. The TiTa alloys are endowed with excellent corrosion resistance by the combination of Ta_2O_5 and TiO_2, which is expected to have popularization and application prospects in the biomedical field.

Professor Zhentao Yu's research group studied a series of TixTa (x = 1, 2, 5, 10, 20, 30, 40, 50, 60, 80 wt.%) biomedical binary Ti alloys. Grade 1 Ti sponge with fine particles and metallurgical grade Ta powders and mixing cloth process were applied, and high-quality alloy ingots with uniform composition and low impurity content were produced by using a triple VAR melting process. Figs. 2.3 and 2.4 show the

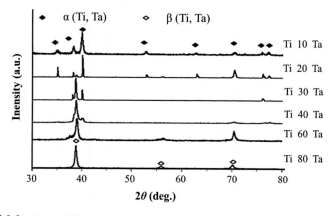

FIGURE 2.3 X-ray diffraction patterns of TiTa alloys.

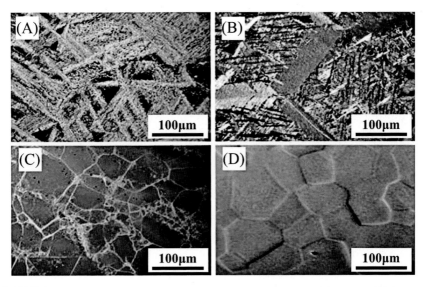

FIGURE 2.4 Optical microstructures of TiTa alloys. (A) Ti10Ta. (B) Ti20Ta. (C) Ti30Ta. (D) Ti60Ta.

X-ray diffraction patterns and metallographic images of the TiTa alloys, respectively. It can be seen that when the Ta content increases, the volume fraction of α phase gradually drops. When the Ta content reaches 60 wt.%, all of the α phase is transformed into the β phase.

2.4.3 TiNbTaZr alloys

Japan Niinomi's research group developed the first biomedical TNTZ metastable β alloy with a lower elastic modulus [7]. Since the TNTZ alloys have high content of Nb, Ta, and other alloying elements that have a much higher melting point and density than metal Ti, by choosing high-quality raw materials (Ti sponge with fine particles, metallurgical grade Ta and Nb powders, and sponge Zr) and using mixed cloth process and triple VAR melting process, they successfully produced high-quality alloy ingots and hot-rolled workpieces with uniform composition and low impurity content, thereby effectively avoiding the macrosegregation of the above alloying elements. The results found that the α phase or ω phase precipitated during aging of this alloy raised the elastic modulus of the alloy, and the elastic modulus decreased if the β and α″ phases were incorporated or large plastic deformation was used to induce the martensite phase transformation and microdefects. The elastic modulus of the TiNbTaZr quaternary β alloy has strong anisotropy, and the elasticity modulus can be close to the level of cortical bone by controlling the rolling direction [25].

2.4.4 TiZr alloys

TiZr alloys have good biocompatibility, moderate strength, and high plasticity and toughness. These are a kind of new type biomedical alloys that are suitable for the design and development of dental products, such as dental implants and denture frameworks. The author's research group successfully designed and prepared a series of new biomedical Ti alloys, TixZr (x = 1, 2, 5, 10, 20, 30, 40, 50, 60 wt.%), with uniform composition and low impurity content using traditional VAR technique. The measured chemical composition of TiZr system alloys is given in Table 2.9 [15].

2.4.5 TiNb alloys

The author's research group has conducted basic research on the composition design, melting, and hot working of TixNb (x = 5, 10, 15, 20, 25 wt.%) biomedical Ti alloys. Fig. 2.5 shows the microstructure of the TiNb alloy bar, from which it can be seen that the size of the precipitates gradually decreases and tends to show a dispersed distribution with increasing of the Nb content [15]. The Ti35Nb alloy has a certain shape memory effect in which was found that when the Nb content increases by 1 at.%, the M_s temperature decreases by 43°C, and the Ti(22−25)Nb alloy has the shape memory effect after the solution treatment at 900°C/30 min. Ti(25.5−27)Nb alloy exhibits superelasticity at room temperature and has a fully recoverable strain of about 2%. After aging at 300°C for 1 hour, fine and dispersed ω phases can be precipitated, thereby enhancing the superelasticity. After cold rolling, the intermediate temperature annealing (600°C/10 min) and aging treatment (300°C/1 h) also enhance the superelasticity of the alloy [26,27].

TABLE 2.9 Chemical composition of TiZr systemic alloys.

Nominal composition	Zr (%)	Fe (%)	Si (%)	C (%)	N (%)	H (%)	O (%)	Ti (%)
Ti1Zr	0.98	0.01	<0.04	0.021	0.007	0.0009	0.078	Bal.
Ti2Zr	1.98	0.01	<0.04	0.019	0.014	0.001	0.082	Bal.
Ti16Zr	16.3	0.02	<0.04	0.015	0.013	0.001	0.09	Bal.
Ti20Zr	20.9	0.01	<0.04	0.014	0.014	0.001	0.084	Bal.
Ti35Zr	35.71	0.03	<0.01	0.008	0.003	0.001	0.086	Bal.
Ti50Zr	48.52	0.05	<0.01	0.01	0.015	0.001	0.081	Bal.
Ti60Zr	41.6	0.02	<0.04	0.008	0.009	0.0037	0.088	Bal.

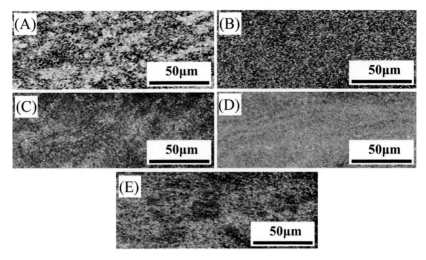

FIGURE 2.5 Microstructure of TiNb alloys. (A) Ti5Nb. (B) Ti10Nb. (C) Ti15Nb. (D) Ti20Nb. (E) Ti25Nb.

2.5 Design and physical metallurgical properties of novel TLM alloy

2.5.1 Design of novel TLM alloy

The selection of alloying elements is very important in the design of novel metastable β biomedical Ti alloys. First of all, the components of the alloys are required to be nontoxic and nonallergenic, and the alloys are required to have high strength, high toughness, low modulus, and excellent cold and hot formability. According to the results of biocompatibility measurements of pure metals and their alloys, it has been found that Ti, Zr, Mo, Sn, Ta, Nb, Pd, and Hf are the additive alloying elements with excellent biocompatibility. Zr, Sn, and Hf are neutral elements, which have a large solid solubility in both α-Ti and β-Ti matrix and have little influence on the point of phase transformation from α to α + β. They can strengthen Ti and have little adverse influence on plasticity, thus ensuring good processing properties of materials. Mo, Nb, Ta, and Pd are β-stabilizing elements, which can be dissolved infinitely in β-Ti matrix and reduce the α/α + β phase transformation temperature. Among them, Mo, Ta, and Nb have strong strengthening effects on Ti and are very beneficial for improving the thermal processing properties of Ti alloys. In addition, Zr, Mo, Ta, and Nb can reduce the elastic modulus of alloys. Nb has little adverse effect on plasticity, even improves the plasticity of alloys, and is also beneficial for the improvement of toughness. Mo can refine the grains and improve the cold and hot formability of alloys. Therefore Zr, Mo, Nb, and Sn should be preferably used as additive elements for ideal novel biomedical metastable β-Ti alloys.

To design and develop new types of near β-Ti alloys with low elastic modulus, high strength, good plasticity and toughness, and relatively low cost for surgical implants, we have selected Zr, Nb, Mo, and Sn with certain ratios and excellent biological and mechanical properties as additives. The molybdenum equivalent of the alloys is kept in the range of 7.2–11.9 to form metastable near β-Ti alloys as listed in Table 2.10. On the basis of the d-electron alloy design theory, the alloy electron orbital parameters in the circular area are selected, where martensite, twins, and dislocations are more generated in the phase diagram, as shown in Fig. 2.6. Then Zr, Sn, Mo, and Nb are selected as the alloying elements, and five pairs of parameters in this area are chosen. Hundreds of TiNbZrMo quaternary system and TiNbZrMoSn pentad systemic alloys have been calculated by the TiCalc program. The positions of the nine new types of β-Ti alloys designed by us are located at the upper right corner of the electron orbital phase diagram. In this region the martensitic transformation of the alloys is prone to occur. The microstructure analysis of these alloys confirms that their micromechanism is the dominant martensitic phase transformation. Finally, on the basis of the low cost of the alloy and good biocompatibility analysis, we have designed a metastable β-Ti alloys TiZrSnMoNb and TiZrMoNb (named TLM and TLE for short, meaning Ti alloy with low modulus or low E) with lower cost and excellent biological and mechanical compatibility.

TABLE 2.10 Alloy design parameters of biomedical β-Ti alloys.

Specimen	Alloy designation	$[Mo]_{Eq}$	$\overline{Bo}$	$\overline{Md}$
1	Ti13Nb13Zr	3.6	2.837	2.483
2	Ti5Zr3Mo15Nb (TLE)	7.2	2.830	2.451
3	Ti5Zr3Mo25Nb	9.9	2.852	2.450
4	Ti5Zr6Mo15Nb	10.2	2.836	2.443
5	Ti3Zr2Sn3Mo25Nb (TLM)	9.9	2.843	2.441
6	Ti1Zr4Sn3Mo25Nb	9.9	2.835	2.431
7	Ti25Nb15Zr	6.9	2.868	2.491
8	Ti25Nb15Zr3Mo	9.9	2.875	2.482
9	Ti10Mo6Zr4Sn3Nb (TB12)	10.9	2.812	2.430

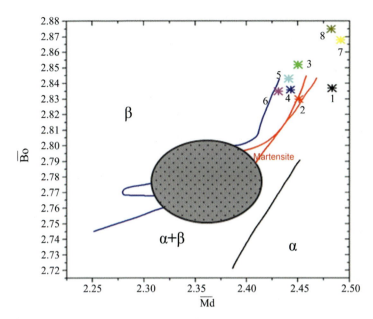

FIGURE 2.6 The position of nine new β-type Ti alloys in the electron orbital diagram.

2.5.2 Smelting and physical metallurgical properties of TLM alloy

For the smelting of small ingots for laboratory research, grade 0 Ti sponge with fine particles, pure Zr bars (99.7%), pure Sn bars (99.9%), pure Mo powders (99.8%), and NbTi master alloy (Nb47Ti) are commonly used as raw materials. First, pure Zr bars, pure Sn bars, and NbTi alloy are made into alloy packages, and pure Mo powders and Ti sponge with fine particles are put into the mixing barrel and fully mixed to ensure that the Mo powders fully penetrate the pores of the Ti sponge. Then the above-mentioned materials are mixed and pressed into alloy electrodes. Nine types of β biomedical TLM Ti alloys are finally obtained by melting the alloy electrodes twice in a consumable electrode vacuum arc furnace. The detection of the chemical composition and observation of the microstructure of the ingots show that the alloys have uniform compositions and very low impurity content and do not have segregations and inclusions. Since the new alloys belong to the metastable β-Ti alloys, it can be found that there are obvious α-phase precipitations with different shapes during the furnace cooling process of the ingots, as shown in Table 2.11 and Fig. 2.7.

The TLM alloy ingots for industrialization are smelted by using consumable electrode VAR technology. First, three types of chip master alloys of Nb47Ti, Ti32Mo, and Ti80Sn are chosen as raw materials. Second, the electrode blocks are pressed by using a 200 × 400 mm mold,

TABLE 2.11 Impurity contents of tested alloy ingots (wt.%).

Alloy number	O	H	C	N	Fe	Si
1	0.07	0.002	0.03	0.014	0.02	<0.04
2	0.08	0.001	0.02	0.020	0.04	<0.04
3	0.08	0.001	0.02	0.020	0.09	<0.04
4	0.08	0.001	0.02	0.018	0.07	<0.04
5	0.10	0.001	0.02	0.023	0.08	<0.04
6	0.10	0.001	0.01	0.013	0.08	<0.04
7	0.08	0.001	0.02	0.020	0.04	<0.04
8	0.11	0.001	0.02	0.015	0.06	<0.04
9	0.08	0.001	0.008	0.004	0.04	<0.04

the bottom and top molds of which are completely symmetrical, contributing to the uniform distribution of pressure. In the meantime, the twice two-way pressing method is adopted to strengthen the density of the electrode blocks with a compactness value of 4.15 g cm^{-3}. To ensure the uniform distribution of the Mb and Mo elements in the ingots, the smelting process of Nb47Ti is used for reference, a large current is used for the first smelting, and the depth of the molten pool is raised, the temperature of the molten pool is increased so that the raw materials with high melting point are fully alloyed. A smaller current is used during the secondary and tertiary smelting to reduce the depth of the molten pool, thereby avoiding the enrichment of the Nb and Mo elements. A larger arc stabilization period is applied to ensure the depth of the center molten pool and reduce the nonmelting blocks to a certain extent.

Fig. 2.8 shows the preparation process route of TLM alloy ingots. Fig. 2.9 shows the electrodes of 145 mm in height prepared by the above-mentioned methods. It can be seen that there are no abnormal phenomena such as delamination, cracking, or porosity from the electrodes and weld seam.

The uniformity of composition of the prepared industrial alloy ingots is given in Tables 2.12 and 2.13. The nominal composition is Ti3Zr2Sn3Mo25Nb, and the target composition is Ti3.1Zr2Sn3.1Mo25Nb. Because of the reasonable selection of alloy and smelting process, the uniformity of the ingot composition is greatly improved. The phase transition point of the TLM alloy measured by the metallographic test is 710°C–720°C, which is 200°C–250°C lower than those of the conventional α and $\alpha + \beta$-Ti alloys.

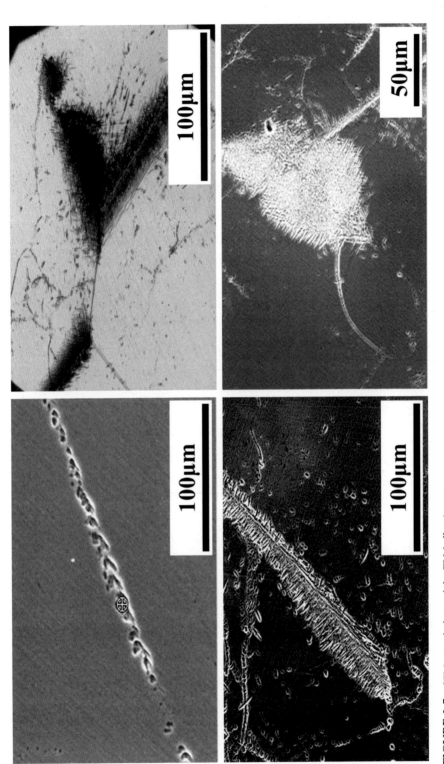

FIGURE 2.7 SEM morphology of the TLM alloy ingot.

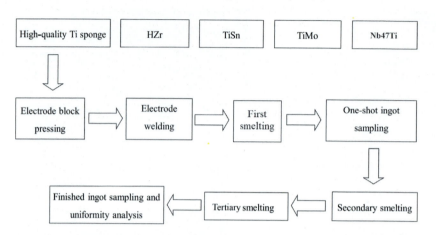

FIGURE 2.8 Preparation of the TLM alloy ingot.

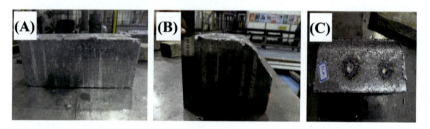

FIGURE 2.9 TLM alloy electrode rod (200 × 400 mm). (A) Length. (B) Cross section. (C) Welding surface.

TABLE 2.12 The uniformity of composition of the TLM alloy ingot (Φ150 mm, 25 kg) (wt.%).

Alloy	Sampling site	Alloying elements				Impurities and interstitial elements				
		Mo	Nb	Sn	Zr	Fe	Si	C	N	H	O
TLM	Top	3.10	25.03	2.03	3.10	0.04	0.04	0.02	0.015	0.001	0.07
	Middle	3.10	24.81	2.10	2.98						
	Bottom	3.04	24.93	1.98	3.17						

TABLE 2.13 The uniformity of composition of the TLM alloy ingot (Φ440 mm, 500 kg) (wt.%).

	Mo	Zr	Sn	Nb
Longitudinal deviation	0.09	0.04	0.10	0.80
Lateral deviation	0.11	0.11	0.09	1.00
Overall deviation	0.12	0.13	0.19	1.40

Different types of β biomedical Ti alloys can be formed by controlling different alloying elements and their proportions, and the formation and evolution of the phase structure and microstructure of the novel near β-Ti alloy TLM are inseparable from the subsequent processing methods and specific technology of smelting, processing, and heat treatment. Then the comprehensive mechanical properties can be investigated and regulated through different microstructures or microscopic deformation mechanisms. In designing and developing of new β biomedical Ti alloys with high strength and low modulus, it has been found that, from a macro perspective, we have to pay attention to the β-stabilizing elements with high melting points and the main influencing factors of their content on the microstructure. From a micro perspective, it is also necessary to focus on the influence of the impurity elements, such as O and N, on the formation of mesophases such as the α', α'', and ω phases. Factors of these mesophases include the structure type, morphology, size, distribution, volume fraction, and microtexture and their effects on the mechanical properties such as the elastic modulus, superelasticity, and shape memory effect of Ti alloys. The comprehensive mechanical properties of the alloy, including strength, modulus, plasticity, and toughness, can be matched well so as to meet the requirements of different surgical implant devices [28−37].

References

[1] Z. Yu, S. Yu, J. Chen, X. Ma, Development and application of novel biomedical titanium alloy materials, Acta Metallurgica Sinica 53 (2017) 90−116.
[2] Z. Yu, S. Yu, M. Zhang, J. Han, X. Ma, Current status and progress in the design, development, and application of new medical titanium alloy materials for surgical implants, Materials China 29 (2010) 35−51.
[3] D. Kuroda, M. Niinomi, M. Morinaga, Y. Kato, T. Yashiro, Design and mechanical properties of new β type titanium alloys for implant materials, Materials Science and Engineering: A 243 (1998) 244−249.
[4] M. Morinaga, The molecular orbital approach and its application to biomedical Ti alloy design, Titanium in Medical and Dental Applications, Woodhead Publishing, 2018, pp. 39−64.
[5] J. Liu, Introduction to Environmental Materials, Metallurgical Industry Press, Beijing, 1999.
[6] Z. Yu, M. Zhang, Y. Tian, J. Cheng, X. Ma, H. Liu, Designation and development of biomedical Ti alloys with finer biomechanical compatibility in long-term surgical implants, Frontiers of Materials Science 8 (2014) 219−229.
[7] M. Geetha, A.K. Singh, K. Muraleedharan, A.K. Gogia, R. Asokamani, Effect of thermomechanical processing on microstructure of a Ti−13Nb−13Zr alloy, Journal of Alloys and Compounds 329 (2001) 264−271.
[8] M. Nakai, M. Niinomi, X. Zhao, X. Zhao, Self-adjustment of Young's modulus in biomedical titanium alloys during orthopaedic operation, Materials Letters 65 (2011) 688−690.

[9] M. Niinomi, M. Nakai, Titanium-based biomaterials for preventing stress shielding between implant devices and bone, International Journal of Biomaterials 2011 (2011) 836587.

[10] X. Zhao, M. Niinomi, M. Nakai, G. Miyamoto, T. Furuhara, Microstructures and mechanical properties of metastable Ti−30Zr−(Cr, Mo) alloys with changeable Young's modulus for spinal fixation applications, Acta Biomaterialia 7 (2011) 3230−3236.

[11] Z. Yu, L. Zhou, M. Fan, S. Yuan, Investigation on near-β Ti alloy Ti-5Zr-3Sn-5Mo-15Nb for surgical implant materials, Materials Science Forum 475−479 (2005) 2353−2358.

[12] Z. Yu, L. Zhou, K. Wang, Research and development of biomedical titanium alloys for surgical implant materials, in: 7th World Biomaterials Congress, Sydney, 2004.

[13] X. Ma, Y. Han, Z. Yu, Q. Sun, J. Niu, S. Yuan, Phase transformation and mechanical properties of TLM titanium alloy for orthopedic implants, Rare Metal Materials and Engineering 41 (2012) 1535−1538.

[14] Z. Yu, L. Zhou, L. Luo, M. Fan, Y. Fu, Investigation on mechanical compatibility matching for biomedical titanium alloys, Key Engineering Materials 288−289 (2005) 595−598.

[15] Z. Yu, S. Yu, J. Cheng, X. Ma, Development and application of novel biomedical titanium alloy materials, Acta Metallurgica Sinica 53 (2017) 1238−1264.

[16] Y. Zhang, L. Zhou, J. Sun, M. Han, P. Ni, D. Chen, et al., Progress of vacuum arc remelting technology of titanium alloys, Rare Metals Letters 27 (2008) 9−14.

[17] L. Zhang, Z. Zhou, H. Chang, X. Xue, Y. Bai, X. Wang, et al., Segregation behavior and preventive measures of β-type titanium alloys with high molybdenum content, The Chinese Journal of Nonferrous Metals 23 (2013) 2206−2212.

[18] W. Lei, Y. Zhao, D. Han, X. Mao, Development of melting technology for titanium and titanium alloys, Materials Reports 30 (2016) 101−106,124.

[19] Z. Yang, Multi-Field Coupling of Titanium Alloy VAR Process and Its Effect on Solidification Behavior, Northwestern Polytechnical University, 2011.

[20] K. Suzuki, N. Fukada, O. Kanou, Optimization of VAR process by applying computational simulation, Ti-2007 Science and Technology, The Japan Institute of Metals, 2007, pp. 155−158.

[21] A. Ballantyne, The development and application of an integrated VAR process model, BHM Berg-und Hüttenmännische Monatshefte 161 (2016) 12−19.

[22] S. Fedotov, T. Chelidze, Y. Kovneristyy, V. Sanadze, Phase transformations during heating of metastable alloys of the Ti−Ta system, Physics of Metals and Metallography (USSR) 62 (1986) 109−113.

[23] Y.L. Zhou, M. Niinomi, T. Akahori, Effects of Ta content on Young's modulus and tensile properties of binary Ti−Ta alloys for biomedical applications, Materials Science and Engineering: A 371 (2004) 283−290.

[24] R. Margevicius, J. Cotton, Stress-assisted transformation in Ti-60 wt pct Ta alloys, Metallurgical and Materials Transactions A 29 (1998) 139−147.

[25] M. Niinomi, M. Nakai, J. Hieda, Development of new metallic alloys for biomedical applications, Acta Biomaterialia 8 (2012) 3888−3903.

[26] T. Inamura, J. Kim, H. Kim, H. Hosoda, K. Wakashima, S. Miyazaki, Composition dependent crystallography of α''-martensite in Ti−Nb-based β-Ti alloy, Philosophical Magazine 87 (2007) 3325−3350.

[27] E. Hamzah, K. Hastuti, J. Hashim, Effect of ageing temperature on the microstructures and mechanical properties of Ti-Nb shape memory alloys, Advanced Materials Research 1024 (2014) 304−307.

[28] Z. Yu, L. Zhou, K. Wang, Design and development of biomedical β-Ti alloys, Rare Metals Letters 23 (2004) 5−10.

References

[29] Z. Yu, L. Zhou, J. Niu, β type titanium alloys used in surgical implant materials, Rare Metal Materials and Engineering 35 (2006) 261−265.

[30] Z. Yu, L. Zhou, Influence of martensitic transformation on mechanical compatibility of biomedical β type titanium alloy TLM, Materials Science and Engineering: A 438 (2006) 391−394.

[31] Z. Yu, L. Zhou, J. Niu, S. Yuan, X. He, Q. Huangfu, et al., Effect of alloy element, process and heat treatment on mechanical properties of β-type biomedical titanium alloy, Chinese Journal of Rare Metals 31 (2007) 416−419.

[32] Z. Yu, Y. Zheng, L. Zhou, B. Wang, J. Niu, Q. Huangfu, et al., Shape memory effect and superelastic property of a novel Ti-3Zr-2Sn-3Mo-15Nb alloy, Rare Metal Materials and Engineering 37 (2008) 1−5.

[33] Z. Yu, G. Wang, X. Ma, Y. Zhang, M. Dargusch, Shape memory characteristics of a near β titanium alloy, Materials Science and Engineering: A 513 (2009) 233−238.

[34] Z. Yu, J. Liu, J. Han, Y. Zhang, Q. Huangfu, X. He, et al., Study on heat treatment and material strengthening of β-type titanium alloy Ti4Zr1Sn3Mo25Nb(TLM), Rare Metal Materials and Engineering 37 (2008) 542−545.

[35] Z. Yu, G. Wang, X. Ma, M. Dargusch, J. Han, S. Yu, Development of biomedical near β-titanium alloys, Materials Science Forum (2009) 303−306.

[36] Z. Yu, X. Ma, S. Yu, M. Zhang, J. Han, C. Liu, Micro-nano technology and latest progress of biomedical titanium alloy, The Chinese Journal of Nonferrous Metals 20 (2010) 1008−1012.

[37] Z. Yu, Y. Zhang, H. Liu, X. Ma, S. Yu, M. Zhang, Effects of alloy elements, processing and heat treatment on mechanical properties of a near β type biomedical titanium alloy TiZrMoNb and microstructure analysis, Rare Metal Materials and Engineering 39 (2010) 1795−1801.

CHAPTER 3

Processing, heat treatment, microstructure, and property evolution of TLM alloy

3.1 Overview of processing and heat treatment of β-Ti alloys

When billeted forging and semifinished products of the β-type Ti alloys are wrought, the process is generally carried out in the β-phase zone because the β-phase with body-centered cubic structure can withstand large thermal deformation, which can fully and uniformly break the coarse grain structure. For semifinished products of metastable β-Ti alloys, such as plates, rods, and forgings, the processing is generally conducted in the α + β-dual-phase zone. At this time, in comparison to the lots of α-phase with dense hexagonal structure abundant in other types of alloys, the metastable β-phase abundant in present Ti alloys has much better intrinsic plasticity. In addition, the Ti alloy materials can be obtained in high quality by controlling heating temperature and deformation amount, especially controlling a certain amount of primary α-phase precipitation.

For any new type of biomedical Ti alloy materials to be designed and finalized, it is vital to meet the needs of subsequent precision processing for different surgical implant devices so that they can be easily processed into conventional materials such as plates, tubes, rods, and strips with different shapes and specifications. The semifinished billets of Ti alloy plates, bars, pipes, and forgings are firstly subjected to large plastic deformation at high temperature (usually above the alloy phase transformation point) so as to fully break the original coarse structures in the as-cast alloy. The commonly used thermal pressure working equipment or methods mainly include free forging, precision forging, and rapid forging. At present, common surgical implants and orthopedic devices are made from commercial Ti alloys. The raw materials, such as plates, tubes, rods, wires, filaments, and foil, used for precision processing are mainly small-sized deep-processed products, which can be obtained by extrusion, rolling, rotary forging, and drawing [1]. The selection of the heating method during the intermediate heat treatment is also very important because Ti is a chemically active metal, which can be easily contaminated by harmful gases such as N_2, O_2, and H_2 at high temperature. To reduce pollution, the current semifinished products of Ti plates and bar stocks in China are mostly heated by using resistance furnaces (muffle furnaces).

According to the alloy composition and content of Nb, Mo, and Zr, the β-phase can be transformed into a metastable phase of α′, α″, or ω after the solution treatment of β-Ti alloys. With further aging treatment at different temperatures and different durations, ω-phase and α-phase with different sizes and shapes can be generated. The temperature range for the occurrence of different phase transitions is wider. The mechanical properties of the alloys rely on the micro- and nanosizes and contents of ω-phase, the metastable β-phase or martensite and other intermediate phases of metastable β-Ti alloys can be maintained at room temperature through solid solution treatment, and then secondary precipitations, such as α, ω, and so on, can be further generated by using aging at low temperature. Thus the required comprehensive mechanical properties can be obtained [2,3]. Moreover, by controlling the appropriate ratio of the primary α-phase and the metastable β-phase as well as the morphology and size of the intermediate phases, such as ω, α′, and α″, the strength, modulus, and plastic toughness of the alloy can achieve a better comprehensive matching [4–13]. Table 3.1 shows the heat treatment and typical microstructure of β-Ti alloys.

3.2 Billets and semifinished products of TLM alloy

Plates and bars of pure Ti and low-alloyed Ti alloy can be mold-forged, rolled, or smelted into flat billets. High-alloyed alloy billets are generally processed by free forging, precision forging, and other equipment. The commonly used billets and semifinished products of Ti3Zr2Sn3Mo25Nb (TLM) alloy generally include forging rods, forging billets, hot rolled bars, hot rolled plates, and extruded tubes, all of which are produced by thermal processing methods, such as billet forging, precision forging, extrusion, hot rolling, or hot rotary forging. The hot processing technology route of a TLM billet is as follows:

Master alloy preparation → All metal materials, press electrodes → Smelting (2–3 times) → Ingot → Ingot surface polishing → Forging (β-forging) → Rectangular type billets → Round O type billets → Bar stock → Performance testing for samples.

TABLE 3.1 Heat treatment and typical microstructure of β-Ti alloys.

Type	Heat treatment	Microstructure
β	Solution treatment above the recrystallization temperature	β-phase
Metastable β	Solution treatment in the β-phase region + rapid cooling (water or oil quenching)	Metastable β-, β'-phase, etc.
	Solution treatment in the β-phase region + rapid cooling + aging	Secondary α-, ω-phase, etc.
	Solution treatment in the β-phase region + air cooling	Metastable β-, β'-, primary α-phase, etc.
	Solution treatment in the β-phase region + air cooling + aging	Primary α-, secondary α-, β-phase, etc.
Near-β	Solution treatment in the β-phase region + rapid cooling (water or oil quenching)	Martensite α'- or α''-phase, etc.
	Solution treatment in the β-phase region + rapid cooling + aging	Primary α-, ω-, and β-phase, etc.
	Solution treatment in the β-phase region + air cooling	Metastable β-, primary α-phase
	Solution treatment in the β-phase region + air cooling + aging	Secondary α-, ω- and β-phase
	Solution treatment in the α + β-phase region + rapid cooling or air cooling	Martensite α'- or α''-phase, primary α- and transforming β-phase, etc.
	Solution treatment in the α + β-phase region + rapid cooling or air cooling + aging	Secondary α- and β-phase, etc.

The forging process has a great influence on the structures and properties of the finished TLM alloy. Generally, the billet forging temperature is 1000°C–1100°C, the precision forging temperature is 820°C ± 50°C, and the rolling temperature is 700°C ± 50°C. Fig. 3.1 shows the metallographic microstructure and mechanical properties of TLM alloy forging bar (Φ98 mm). Too high a forging temperature will cause coarsening of the structure. Therefore it is extremely important to select an appropriate forging temperature. Fig. 3.2 shows the metallographic microstructure of a Φ35 mm bar. It can be seen that there is a large amount of plastic deformation martensite in the edge structure of the bar and that the amount of martensite gradually decreases from the edge to the center of the specimen.

58   3. Processing, heat treatment, microstructure, and property evolution of TLM alloy

Yield strength $R_{0.2}$	Tensile strength R_m	A, %	Z, %
357	576	41	80
394	611	35.5	80

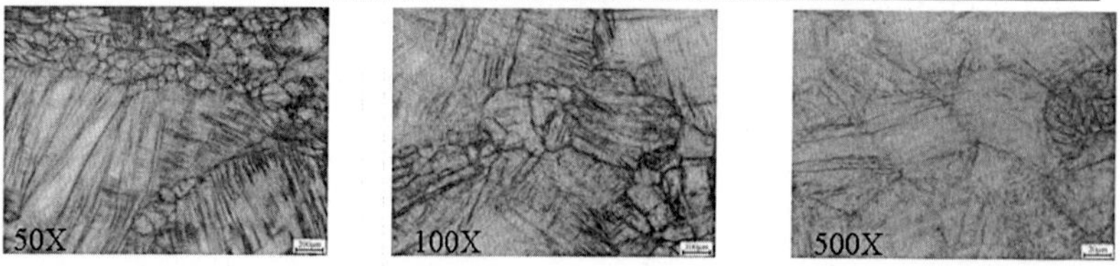

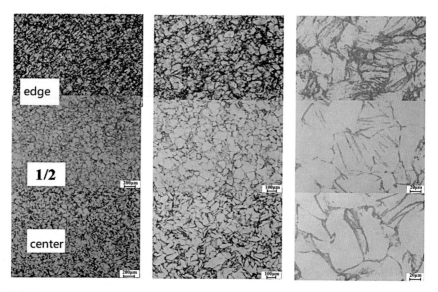

FIGURE 3.1 Metallographic structure and mechanical properties of TLM Ti alloy forging rod (Φ98 mm).

FIGURE 3.2 Metallographic structure of TLM alloy forging rod (Φ35 mm).

The high-temperature tensile test results of TLM alloy are shown in Fig. 3.3. It can be seen that the tensile strength of the alloy drops below 100 MPa and the deformation resistance significantly decreases when the testing temperature is higher than 700°C. These results indicate that the alloy has good thermal processing performance, which is convenient for the thermal processing of ingots, plates, bars, and so on.

3.3 Plates and strips of TLM alloy

TLM Ti alloy plates are processed in the β-phase zone, the heating temperature is 900°C−1000°C, and the hot rolling deformation rates are 70%−90%.

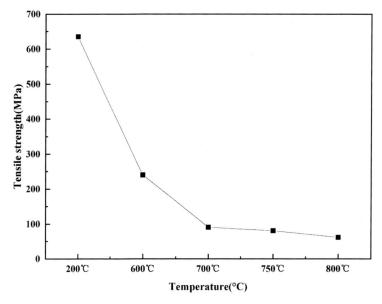

FIGURE 3.3   Tensile strength–temperature curve of TLM alloys.

When the processing is conducted in the $\alpha + \beta$-phase zone, the hot rolling temperature is 600°C–700°C and the hot rolling deformation rates are 50%–70%. Plates that are 10, 5, and 2 mm in thickness can be produced by hot rolling. During the cold rolling process, the deformation rates should be controlled at 20%–40%, and the rolling direction of the plate should be reversed during each working pass. The processing procedures for plates are as follows:

TLM cast ingot → Forging → Blank → Hot rolling → Plates → Surface dressing, heat treatment → Cold rolling → Plates → Heat treatment → Finished sheet → Performance testing

The microstructure of hot rolled Ti alloy plates subjected to different heat treatment is shown in Fig. 3.4. It can be seen that all the alloy plates consist of equiaxial grains, and the average grain size is between 8 and 52 μm after solution treatment at 710°C–820°C, as shown in Fig. 3.4A–C. The new second phase is precipitated after solid solution aging, that is, ω-phase newly formed during low-temperature aging, whereas the α-second phase appears during aging at 510°C, which is consistent with the results of previous studies [14,15]. However, the difference is that the size of the α-phase is much smaller than that of the reported counterpart, which has not yet grown into large crystal grains with strip shape, owing to the initial stage of formation

The mechanical properties of cold rolled TLM Ti alloy sheet are shown in Table 3.2. After TLM alloy is deformed by cold rolling, it can

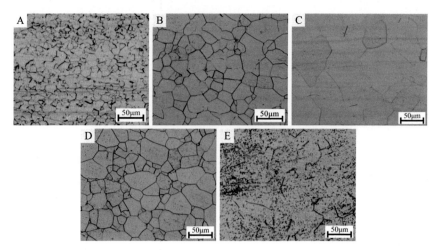

FIGURE 3.4 Microstructure of TLM alloy plates under different heat treatments. (A) 680°C/1 h, AC. (B) 750°C/1 h, AC. (C) 820°C/1 h, AC. (D) 750°C/1 h, AC + 350°C /1 h, AC. (E) 750°C/1 h, AC + 510°C/1 h, AC. *Source: data from X. Ma, Z. Yu, J. Niu, S. Yu, J. Cheng, Effect of heat treatment on superelasticity in Ti-3Zr-2Sn-3Mo-25Nb alloy, Rare Metal Materials and Engineering. 45 (2016) 1588–1592.*

TABLE 3.2 Mechanical properties of TLM alloy cold rolled sheet (1 mm in thickness).

Sample	R_m (MPa)	R_p (MPa)	A (%)	E (GPa)	Direction
1	980	895	11.5	78.0	Rolling direction
	975	890	13.0	83.0	
2	935	850	14.5	89.0	Vertical rolling direction
	935	850	15.0	83.2	

be seen that the grain deformation direction and cold rolling deformation direction will be more consistent with the further increase in the cold deformation, and there is no obvious anisotropy in the transverse and longitudinal directions of the plate.

Fig. 3.5 shows the heat treatment parameters of the TLM sheet treated under solid solution at 650°C, 710°C, 750°C, and 800°C for 1 hour and then subsequent water cooled, followed by aging treatment at 380°C, 450°C, and 510°C and then a double-stage aging process. During the double-stage aging process, the specimens were held at 380°C for 4 hours, then directly heated in the furnace to 450°C, and finally taken out.

Fig. 3.6 shows the X-ray diffraction (XRD) spectra of the cold rolled sheet under different heat treatment conditions. The figure shows that in the cold

3.3 Plates and strips of TLM alloy

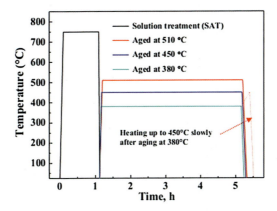

FIGURE 3.5 Heat treatment parameters of TLM plate.

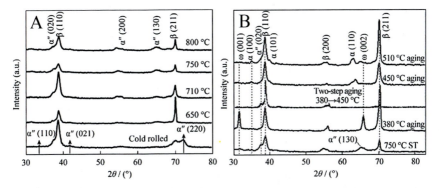

FIGURE 3.6 X-ray diffraction spectra of TLM alloy plate after different heat treatment. (A) Solution treated at 650, 710, 750, and 800°C for 1 h, respectively. (B) Solution treated at 750°C and then aged at 380, 450, and 510°C for 4 h, respectively. "Two-step aging 380 → 450°C" indicating a post-aging process of heating up to 450°C at 5°C min^{-1} after aged at 380°C. Source: data from X. Ma, H. Niu, Z. Yu, S. Yu, C. Wang, Microstructural adjustments and mechanical properties of a cold-rolled biomedical near β − Ti alloy sheet, Rare Metals 37 (2018) 846–851.

rolling state, the β-phase and the orthorhombic α″-martensite coexist in the alloy. The formation of the orthorhombic α″-martensite is caused mainly by the stress-induced phase transformation during the cold rolling process. After solution treatment at 650°C for 1 hour or higher temperature, the stress-induced α″-martensite completely disappeared, and some new α″-martensite peaks appeared, indicating that the β-type TLM alloy after rapid quenching from high temperature can lead to the transformation from β- to α″-martensite [16−18]. Fig. 3.6B shows the XRD patterns of the alloy after solid solution and aging. Compared with the solid solution state, almost all the α″-phases are eliminated after aging at 380°C for 4 hours, and the ω-phase of the hexagonal structure is generated. The ω-phase is a fairly hard and brittle phase, which will reduce the plasticity of biomedical Ti materials. Therefore the samples were further heated to 450°C in the furnace at a heating rate of 5°C min^{-1}, resulting in the disappearance of ω-phase and reoccurrence of α″-phase. In contrast, after aging at 450°C and 510°C for 4 hours, the ω-phase and α″-martensite both disappeared, and only the α-phase was formed. This proves that after aging at a higher temperature but below the β-phase transformation point, the α″-martensite can undergo reversible transformation, namely α″ → β-phase [19].

The optical images of cold rolled TLM alloy sheet after different heat treatments are shown in Fig. 3.7. The crystal grain size in the samples after solid solution and aging treatment are both 20 and 30 μm. However, it is difficult to detect the α″-phase in the XRD spectra of the specimens after two-stage aging, as shown in Fig. 3.7A and C, which is mainly because of the small size of the precipitation. However, some coarse α-phase particles can be found at the grain boundaries in the two-stage aged samples. In addition, there are no ω-phase and α-phase in the alloys after aging at 380°C and 450°C. As the aging temperature is increased to 510°C, the α-particles continue to coarsen.

The transmission electron microscope (TEM) morphologies of the TLM alloy plate after different heat treatments are shown in Fig. 3.8. The fine α″-martensite in samples for solid solution treatment is further confirmed, as shown in Fig. 3.8A. These α″-martensites are formed in β-crystals and

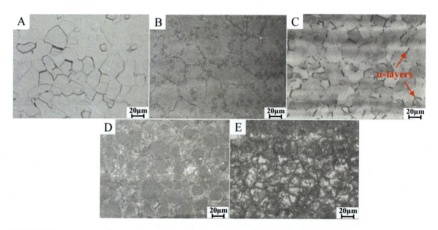

FIGURE 3.7 Optical images of cold rolled TLM alloy sheet after different heat treatments. (A) Solution treated at 750°C, and then (B) aged at 380°C, (C) two—step aged at 380 → 450°C, (D) aged at 450°C, and (E) aged 510°C for 4 h, respectively. *Source: data from X. Ma, H. Niu, Z. Yu, S. Yu, C. Wang, Microstructural adjustments and mechanical properties of a cold-rolled biomedical near β − Ti alloy sheet, Rare Metals 37 (2018) 846–851.*

3.3 Plates and strips of TLM alloy

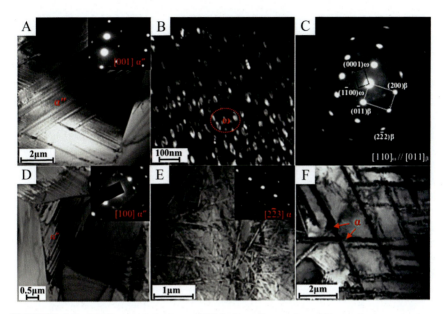

FIGURE 3.8 TEM morphologies of TLM alloy plates after different heat treatments. (A) Solution treated at 750°C and then (B) aged at 380°C, (D) two–step aged at 380 → 450°C, (E) aged at 450°C, and (F) aged at 510°C, followed by air cooling, respectively. (C) Corresponding selected area diffraction spots of ω precipitates and β matrix. *Source: data from X. Ma, H. Niu, Z. Yu, S. Yu, C. Wang, Microstructural adjustments and mechanical properties of a cold-rolled biomedical near β − Ti alloy sheet, Rare Metals 37 (2018) 846–851.*

transformed β-crystals. For the metastable β-Ti alloy, owing to the low thermal stability of the β-phase, it is easy to form α″-martensitic variants after high-temperature quenching in the β-phase region. However, owing to the relatively high content of β-stability element in the TLM alloy, quenching limits the formation of α″-martensite. In Fig. 3.8B, the ellipsoidal ω-phase is formed during the aging process at 380°C, and its size is 15–40 nm. At the same time, the orientation relationship between ω-phase and β-phase accords with $(0\,0\,0\,1)_\omega //(1\,\bar{1}\,1)_\beta, (1\,\bar{1}\,0\,0)_\omega //(2\,1\,\bar{1})_\beta$ and $[1\,1\,\bar{2}\,0]_\omega //[0\,1\,1]_\beta$. The diffraction spot of ω-phase is not found in the selected area electron diffraction images, as shown in Fig. 3.8C, which may be because the size of ω-phase is too small to be detected. Fig. 3.8D shows that α″-martensite reappears during the aging process as the temperature is increased from 380°C to 450°C, but a small amount of fine and long α″ is found only in certain β-grains. After heat treatment at 450°C and 510°C for 4 hours, only the α-phase precipitates can be found, as shown in Fig. 3.8E and F. As the temperature increases, the density of α-phase increases, which is consistent with the observations of XRD and OM analysis, but α-phase has been significantly coarsened at this time, with an average size ranging from 30 to 100 nm.

Fig. 3.9 shows the tensile mechanical properties of TLM alloy sheets at room temperature after different heat treatments. The minimum yield strength of the sample treated at 750°C is 340 MPa, the minimum elastic modulus is 54 GPa, and the elongation is 39%. Although the orthorhombic α″-phase has rare slip systems, its strength and hardness are low, and the Young's modulus is close to that of β-phase. At the same time, the low Young's modulus and high plasticity after solution treatment are attributed to the softer β-matrix phase. The precipitation of high-density ω-nanoparticles after aging at 380°C leads to the high strength of the alloy. The maximum yield strength reaches 1140 MPa, but the elongation is only 5%. When the aging temperature slowly rises from 380°C to 450°C, the ω-phase dissolves slowly, the elongation rate reaches 32%, and the yield strength is 408 MPa, which is caused by the metastable β-phase.

To be an ideal surgical implanting material, the alloy needs good comprehensive mechanical properties such as high strength, low modulus, and high plasticity. After aging at 450°C, a large number of fine needle-like α-phase precipitate in parent β-phase, which help the alloy to achieve high yield strength (770 MPa), moderate elastic modulus (75 GPa), and good elongation (15%). In addition, aging at 510°C coarsens α-phase, owing to the strong growth driving force of α-phase rather than a nucleation driving force, which leads to a decrease in strength and elastic modulus and an increase in plasticity. Therefore aging at 450°C–510°C is more suitable for processing TLM Ti plates. The mechanical properties and photos of related TLM alloy plates are shown in Table 3.3 and Fig. 3.10, respectively.

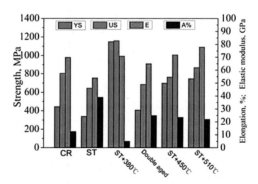

FIGURE 3.9 Tensile mechanical properties at room temperature of TLM alloy plates after different heat treatments. *Source: data from X. Ma, H. Niu, Z. Yu, S. Yu, C. Wang, Microstructural adjustments and mechanical properties of a cold-rolled biomedical near β − Ti alloy sheet, Rare Metals 37 (2018) 846−851.*

TABLE 3.3 Mechanical properties of TLM alloy plates at room temperature.

Plates (mm)	R_m (MPa)	R_p (MPa)	A (%)	Z (%)	Bend angle, α (degrees)
0.8–2	≥ 850	≥ 730	≥ 10	≥ 30	40
2–5	≥ 850	≥ 730	≥ 10	≥ 30	30
5–10	≥ 900	≥ 835	≥ 10	≥ 30	–

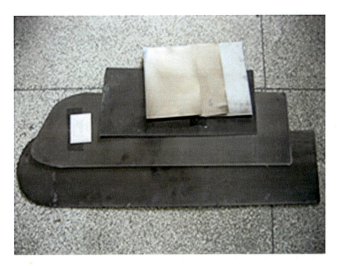

FIGURE 3.10 Photo of TLM alloy sheets.

3.4 Bars and rods of TLM alloy

When TLM alloy bars or rods are processed in the β-phase region, a heating temperature of 900°C–1000°C is selected, and the hot rolling deformation rates are ≤ 80%. When the alloy is processed in the α + β-phase region, a hot rolling temperature of 600°C–700°C is selected, and the heat deformation rates are ≤ 70%. TLM alloy bars can be easily processed to obtain various bar products by commonly used hot rolling, hot rotary swaging, hot drawing, and cold drawing methods. The processing route is as follows:

Ingot→Forging→Bar blank→Hot rolling (β-phase region and α + β-phase region)→Rod (Φ12 and Φ8 mm)→Heat treatment→Rod (Φ12 and Φ8 mm)→Multimode rotary swaging or drawing→Rod→Heat treatment→Finished Rod→Performance testing.

TLM alloys possess excellent processing plastic deformation ability and comprehensive mechanical properties matching. Fig. 3.11 shows photos of typical samples of TLM alloy rods, and Tables 3.4 and 3.5 show the related

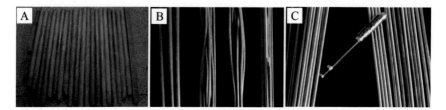

FIGURE 3.11 Pictures of typical TLM alloy rods. (A) Hot forged and then (B) hot rolled followed by (C) heat treatment.

TABLE 3.4 Effect of rolling process and heat treatment on mechanical properties of TLM alloy rods.

E (GPa)	R_m (MPa)	R_p (MPa)	A (%)	Z (%)	Processing information
66	783	413	18	56	Hot rolling in β-phase area for Φ12-mm rod from 5-kg ingot
80	993	863	13	—	Hot rolling in α + β-phase area for Φ8-mm rod from 5-kg ingot
54	690	340	19	81	Hot rolling in β-phase area for Φ8-mm rod from 25-kg ingot
52	823	443	20	85	Hot rolling in α + β-phase area for Φ8-mm rod from 25-kg ingot
92	645	340	39	—	750°C/1 h
81	1270	—	6.0	38	750°C/30 min + 300°C/8 h
71	1160	1150	13	49	750°C/30 min + 386°C/8 h
54	765	700	24	76	750°C/30 min + 480°C/8 h
78	868	748	22	—	750°C/30 min + 510°C/8 h

processing information, heat treatment conditions, and typical mechanical properties. Compared with rolling in the β-phase region, the materials that were rolled in the dual-phase region have higher strength, which is related to fine grains and fine needle martensite obtained by solution quenching followed rolling. TLM Ti alloys possess a low elastic modulus, a wide strength range, and high elongation after heat treatment, which can meet the application requirements of different surgical implants.

Fig. 3.12A shows the metallographic image of a TLM alloy rod sample (Φ12 mm) hot rolled in the β-phase region. It can be seen that after high-temperature deformation in the β-phase area, the original phase in the alloy is fully broken, and the obvious processing streamline remains.

TABLE 3.5 Mechanical properties of typical TLM alloy products (from 250-kg industrial ingot).

Materials	R_m (MPa)	R_p (MPa)	A_5 (%)	Z (%)	E (GPa)	Treatment process
Φ90 Hot forging rod	930	895	12.5	40.5	81.0	RP1 + ST3 + A1
	970	935	11.0	39.0	81.3	
Φ35 Hot forging rod	950	845	16.5	68.5	78.9	RP1 + ST3 + A1
	950	835	15.5	61.5	81.1	
Φ15 Hot rolled rod	945	755	17.0	64.0	79.9	RP1 + ST3 + A1
	925	790	18.0	66.0	76.2	
Φ12 hot rolled rod	940	895	20.5	73.5	79	RP1 + ST3 + A1
	950	895	19.5	73.0	79	
Φ8 Hot rolled rod	985	850	15.0	70.0	87.5	RP1 + ST3 + A1
	900	750	17.0	71.0	89.2	

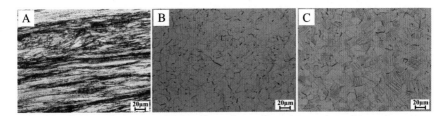

FIGURE 3.12 Microstructure of hot rolled rod samples in the β-phase area of TLM alloy. (A) As-processed. (B) Solid solution treated. (C) Solid solution and aging treatment.

However, owing to the low β-phase transition point of the novel alloy, there are still many broken β-grains and recrystallization during the wrought process, leading to the precipitation of α-phase during cooling. As a result, the alloy still has high strength and plasticity in the processed state, which is why direct aging can be selected to further improve the mechanical properties of the alloy. To improve the material properties, including strength, the alloy should be further aged. The metallographic image of the hot rolled alloy rod sample (Φ12 mm) in β-phase region followed by solution treatment is shown in Fig. 3.12B. After solid solution treatment in the α + β-phase area (680°C), the grains of TLM alloy are in the recovery and recrystallization stage, so the grain size is small and the obvious equiaxed transformation is absent, a small number of wrought traces can be observed, and a small amount of primary α-phase precipitates is discovered in air cooling. After solid solution treatment in the phase β region (750°C), TLM alloy mainly exhibits an equiaxed β-microstructure. Fig. 3.12C shows the metallographic microstructure of a TLM hot rolled bar sample (Φ12 mm) followed by solution treatment and aging treatment. It can be seen that during aging treatment, the metastable β-phase produced by solid solution treatment begins to decompose, and the uniformly distributed secondary α-phase with point and needle shape gradually precipitates in the metastable β-phase matrix, resulting in better comprehensive mechanical properties of TLM alloy materials.

Fig. 3.13 shows the microstructure of TLM alloy after different solid solution treatment and water cooling. It can be seen that after solid solution treatment at the temperature below the phase transformation point, the alloy shows a two-state microstructure. The equiaxed β-microstructure with fine grains was obtained by solid solution treated at 750°C. When the solution temperature rises to 950°C, the β-grain grows rapidly, and there are traces of sunken structure in the matrix, which is mainly to the result of the melting of Sn with a low melting point during the solid solution and subsequently rapid cooling process. Fig. 3.14 shows the microstructure of TLM alloy with different cooling rates after holding at 950°C. It can be seen that there are a large number of fluid concave microstructures under the four cooling methods, but no obvious martensitic transformation was found. Therefore to obtain fine equiaxed β-crystals, the solid solution treatment process of TLM alloy can be chosen to be heat treated at 750°C for 30–60 minutes and then water cooled at room temperature.

Table 3.6 shows tensile mechanical properties of TLM alloy at room temperature for a Φ12 mm rod after hot rolling in the β-phase region and different solid solution and aging treatments. Table 3.7 shows tensile mechanical properties of a Φ8 mm rod after hot rolling in the α + β-phase region and different solid solution and aging treatments. It can be seen that the hot rolling processes in the two-phase region are both reasonable and feasible, indicating that the novel alloy has excellent processing workability [20]. During solid solution heat treatment the cooling methods (water quenching and air cooling) have little influence on the properties of TLM alloy materials, so

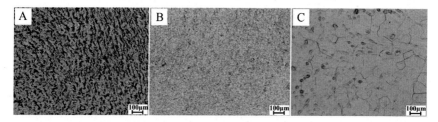

FIGURE 3.13 The microstructure of TLM alloy solid solution treated at different temperatures after water cooling. (A) 650°C. (B) 750°C. (C) 950°C.

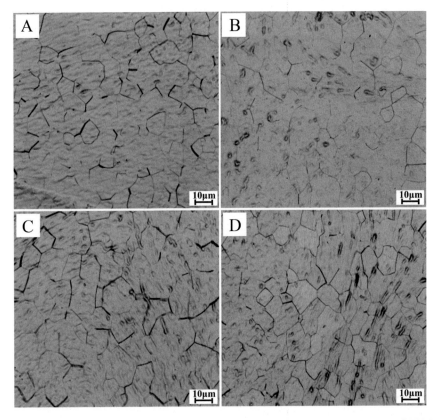

FIGURE 3.14 The influence of four cooling methods on the microstructure of TLM alloy. (A) 23°C. (B) Water quenching. (C) −80°C, (D) −196°C.

they can be adopted according to practical requirements and needs. Hence the comprehensive mechanical properties of TLM alloy materials treated by solid solution in the $\alpha + \beta$-phase region and aging at low temperature are generally better than those of their counterparts with solid solution in β-phase region and aging at high temperature. Better comprehensive mechanical properties can also be obtained by directly aging the hot rolled samples in the β-phase region, which is especially effective for improving the strength of TLM alloy materials. In carrying out solid solution aging treatment, prolonging the aging time has little effect on improving the properties of TLM alloy materials and even leads to the degradation of the properties of the materials. According to different TLM rods, the heat treatment during short duration (4−6 hours) is also generally selected.

TLM alloy rods can also be processed by cold rotary swaging. The cross-sectional metallographic microstructure of the alloy is shown in Fig. 3.15, revealing a typical marbled microstructure with fine fibrous

TABLE 3.6 Tensile mechanical properties of TLM alloy at room temperature (samples were taken from rods (Φ12 mm) hot rolled in the β-phase region).

Alloy	R_m (MPa)	R_p (MPa)	A (%)	Z (%)	E (GPa)	Heat treatment
Ti15Mo5Zr3Al (Japan)	882–975	870–968	25	48	75	ST
	1099–1312	1087–1284	11	43	88–113	STA
Ti29Nb13Ta5Zr (Japan)	911	864	13	–	80	STA
Ti13Nb13Zr (United States)	1030	900	–	–	79	ST
	973–1037	836–908	10–16	27–53	79–84	STA
Ti35Nb5Ta7Zr (United States)	597	547	19	68	55	ST
	1070	976	–	–	–	STA
Ti16Nb10Hf (United States)	851	736	10	–	81	ST
TLM (China)	775–790	390–435	15–21	56	57–76	Hot rolled
	620–760	310–365	21–39	74–83	58–73	ST
	700–1010	560–960	17–22	67–72	62–84	STA
	1020–1060	985–1020	15–18	70–77	68–89	DA

TABLE 3.7 Tensile mechanical properties of TLM alloy at room temperature (samples were taken from rods (Φ8 mm) by hot rolled in α + β-phase region).

Processes	R_m (MPa)	R_p (MPa)	A (%)	E (GPa)
Hot rolled	965–1020	825–900	13	76.2–83
Solid solution	660–1080	385–1050	7.7–29	69–121.4
Aging	750–1090	680–985	12–25	77.5–109

interwoven texture. This kind of microstructure is generated by a large number of nanoscale lattice disturbances in TLM alloy, which might gradually turn into a large number of discontinuous staggered deformations or dislocation-free deformations.

Table 3.8 shows the mechanical properties of TLM alloy after different cold rotary swaging processes. It can be seen that when the deformation rate is 20%–40%, the strength of the novel alloy increases, and the plasticity decreases with the increase of cold deformation. When the cold working rate reaches 60%, the strength and plasticity change slowly. The tensile strength can reach 1250 MPa, and the elongation is

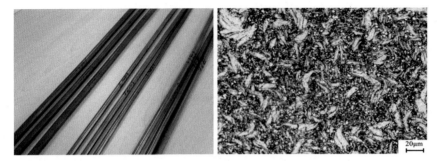

FIGURE 3.15 The cross-sectional morphology of cold rotary forged TLM alloy rods.

TABLE 3.8 Mechanical properties of TLM alloy after different cold forging process.

Cold reduction (%)	R_m (MPa)	R_p (MPa)	A (%)
0	788	700	18
20	865	781	15
40	1080	890	13
60	1170	950	10
80	1250	1080	8

kept at about 8% when the cold deformation rate reaches 80%, so the work hardening of TLM alloy is also obvious. However, with the increase of cold deformation, the yield strength and tensile strength show little difference, which is basically consistent with the strength changes of many metastable or near β-Ti alloys.

3.5 Tubes of TLM alloy

The rod billets of TLM alloy are processed in the β-phase region at a heating temperature of 900°C–1000°C and hot rolling deformation of 80% or less. Then TLM alloy rod billets can be easily processed to prepare various tube products after extrusion, hot rolling, and cold rolling. During cogging rolling (two-roller bending) and finishing rolling (three-roller bending), the accumulative deformation rates are ≤70% and ≤60%, respectively. The relevant tube processing route is as follows:

Ingot→Forging→Bar blank→Machine processing, hole drilling, copper cladding→Hollow billet→Extrusion→Tube billet→Hot rolling→Cold rolling→Heat treatment→Tube finishing→Performance test.

3.5.1 Hot extrusion tube of TLM alloy

After machining, drilling, and copper cladding, the TLM alloy rod billet (Φ98 mm) is extruded into tubes (Φ38 × 7 mm) by a 1500 T horizontal extruder, as shown in Fig. 3.16. Fig. 3.17 shows the cross-sectional metallographic microstructure of TLM alloy tube after hot extrusion above the β-phase region. It can be seen that the microstructure consists of nearly equiaxial grains with an average grain size of about 15 μm. TLM alloy tubes possess good plasticity and cold working

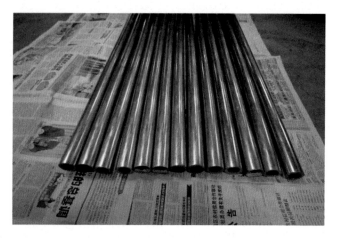

FIGURE 3.16   Extruded tube billets of TLM alloy.

FIGURE 3.17   Metallography of a TLM alloy tube.

TABLE 3.9 Mechanical properties of extruded tube of TLM alloy.

Tube size	R_m (MPa)	R_P (MPa)	A (%)
Φ38 × 7 mm	636	514	42.5

TABLE 3.10 Typical mechanical properties of TLM alloy tubes.

Tubes (mm)	Heat treatment	R_m (MPa)	R_P (MPa)	E (GPa)	A (%)
Φ10.9 × 1.1	510°C/1 h, AC	808	541	62.0	17
	750°C/1 h, FC	776	510	68.3	25
	750°C/1 h, AC + 510°C/4 h, AC	606	270	73.2	37
Φ8.3 × 0.7	510°C/1 h, AC	858	651	60.1	16
	750°C/1 h, FC	740	668	84.3	29
	750°C/1 h, AC + 510°C/4 h, AC	612	271	71.5	47
Φ6 × 0.5	As-rolled	630	465	75.9	51
	510°C/1 h, AC	588	276	67.3	58
	680°C/1 h, FC	809	781	78.6	27
	510°C/1 h, AC	886	639	63.4	25
	680°C/1 h, AC + 510°C/4 h, AC	666	295	71.0	15
	750°C/1 h, AC + 510°C/4 h, AC	714	368	68.6	28

performance after being extruded in the β-phase region, as shown in Table 3.9.

3.5.2 Cold rolled tube of TLM alloy

The tubes with high quality and different specification can be successfully prepared successively by rolling mills LG30, LD15, and LD8. During the fabrication the accumulated deformation rates for cogging rolling and finishing rolling stages are ≤70% and ≤60%, respectively, and single-pass deformation rates is in the range from 20% to 40%, and the solid solution treatment temperature 650°C–800°C and aging treatment temperature 510°C are set, respectively. The room temperature tensile properties of TLM alloy tubes are shown in Table 3.10.

3.5.3 Relationship among processing, microstructure, and properties of TLM alloy tubes

1. Effect of processing deformation on the mechanical properties of TLM tubes

Before testing for tensile mechanical properties, the TLM alloy tubes (Φ12 × 1.2 mm) was cold rolled with deformation rates of 15%, 28%, 34%, and 40%. The corresponding relationship between the processing deformation rates and mechanical properties of the tubes is shown in Fig. 3.18.

It can be seen from Fig. 3.18 that when the deforming rates is between 15% and 28%, the plasticity is very sensitive to deformation hardening and drops sharply. When the deforming rate is between 28% and 35%, the strength decreases slightly, the elongation increases, and the anisotropy among internal grains decreases, which is beneficial to deformation. When the deforming rate is higher than 35%, the yield strength decreases and the elongation continues to increase, which results from the martensite phase transformation of TLM alloy.

2. Effect of the Q value on the mechanical properties of TLM tubes

The Q value is the ratio between the relative wall reduction and the relative diameter reduction. Controlling the Q value can change

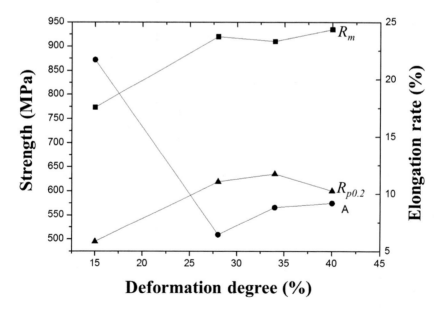

FIGURE 3.18 The relationship between processing deformation and mechanical properties of TLM alloy tubes.

the texture orientation of materials, and then the mechanical properties of tubes can be optimized through regulating the textures. It has been proved that the radial texture distributed along the cross section of tubes is helpful to improve the strength and plasticity, and the circumferential texture is beneficial to improve the processing performance [21]. It can be seen from Fig. 3.19 that when the Q values of a near β-alloy tube change from 0.86 to 2.62, the strength and plasticity decrease with the increase in Q value. This phenomenon may indicate that the radial texture decreases with the increase in Q value. Of course, it also relates to the size effect of the tubes with thinner wall and smaller diameter, so this near-β-TLM alloy should not be processed with large Q values ($Q > 2$).

3. Effect of annealing temperature on the mechanical properties of TLM tubes

TLM alloy tube samples that were Φ8 mm in diameter were treated with 1 hour of solid solution treatment at 680°C, 715°C, 750°C, and 820°C, and the samples were cooled by water quenching (WQ), air cooling (AC), and furnace cooling (FC). The tensile property test results of the samples are shown in Fig. 3.20. It can be seen that the higher the solid solution temperature is, the lower the strength and the better the plasticity of the TLM tubes.

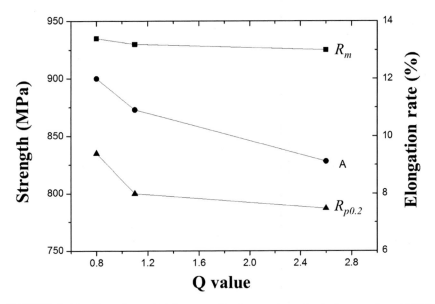

FIGURE 3.19 The relationship between Q values and mechanical properties of TLM alloy tubes.

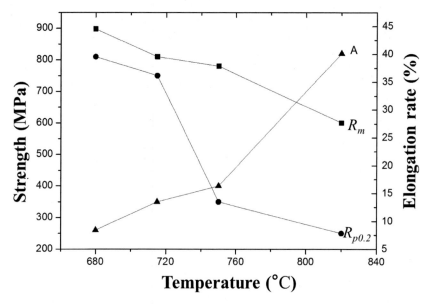

FIGURE 3.20 Relationship between annealing temperature and TLM alloy pipe properties.

The ratio between yield strength and tensile strength (R_p/R_m) is an important indicator to judge the plasticity of metal materials, which is one of the important bases for developing metal plastic processing craft or technology. In general, the difference between the yield strength (R_p) and the tensile strength (R_m) of Ti and Ti alloys is relatively small, which means that the R_p/R_m value is high, generally more than 80%, while the R_p/R_m values of many Ti alloys with medium or high strength exceed 95%, which leads to relatively poor plasticity [22]. Fig. 3.21 shows the curve of the effect of different heat treatment temperatures on the R_p/R_m values of a TLM alloy tube. It can be seen from Fig. 3.21 that with the increase in solid solution temperature, the change of R_p/R_m values is consistent with the plastic variation, resulting in obvious softening or decrease in yield strength. Above the phase transformation point, the values of R_p/R_m are less than 60%, which is much smaller than that of industrial Ti alloys, demonstrating that TLM alloy is particularly suitable for cold deforming and processing.

4. Effect of annealing temperature on the metallographic microstructure

Fig. 3.22 shows the metallographic microstructure of the TLM alloy tube after solid solution treatment at different temperatures. It can be seen that in the tube specimen after solid solution at the temperature below the phase transition point (680°C) and air cooling, the microstructure consists mainly of needle-like primary α_p-phase and

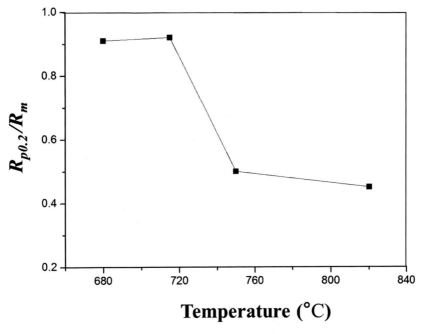

FIGURE 3.21 Effect of heat treatment temperatures on the $R_{p0.2}/R_m$ value of a TLM alloy tube.

$\beta_{transition}$-phase, retaining most of the processing microstructure, and the alloy is in the recovery stage. The working hardening effect has not been eliminated, and the strength is high while the plasticity is poor. After solid solution treatment at the temperature near the phase transition point (715°C), fine recrystallized grains appeared in the microstructure. At this time, the internal defect density decreased, and the dislocation mobility was strong, leading to the decreased strength and the recovered plasticity. After solid solution at 750°C and air cooling, the microstructure consists of a large number of metastable β-phase and a small amount of fine primary α_p-phase, and recrystallization with grain refinement is obvious. After solid solution at 820°C and air cooling, the microstructure presents typical metastable β-phase equiaxial microstructure due to grain recrystallization and growth, and the plasticity of alloy reaches more than 40%, showing good workability.

3.6 TLM alloy products with special specifications

Because of the excellent cold working plasticity and toughness of TLM alloys, they can be easily processed for different specific

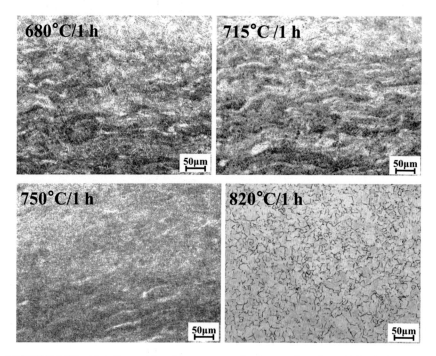

FIGURE 3.22 Metallographic microstructure of tube samples after solid solution treatment at different temperatures.

materials with small size and special shape, that is, special materials with the characteristics of small dimensions or miniaturization, a special process or method, professionalization, and multipurpose applications, meeting the needs of special devices and products in different biomedical fields.

3.6.1 TLM alloy tubes with small diameters and thin walls

When the diameter of the metal tube is close to the critical working size (Φ3 mm) of the rolling mill, the traditional rolling method cannot accomplish its processing. As a result of this concern, we adopted long-core mandrel drawing and hollow-core drawing, in which the drawing deformation is controlled to be 10%–30% for each processing pass, and the total drawing deformation rates is 30%–50%. During the drawing processes, the lubrication was realized by the specific precoating technology [23], and the vacuum heat treatment was conducted at 700°C–800°C for 1 hour. As a result, the smaller and thinner TLM alloy tubes had high quality, including excellent comprehensive mechanical properties, smooth surface, and high-dimensional accuracy, by controlling the factors such as pass deformation ε, Q value, contractile strain ratio (CSR) value, grain sizes, and orientation texture. By using the abovementioned processing methods, tubes with the smallest diameter of 0.8 mm and wall thickness of 0.1 mm can be successfully produced [24], as shown in Fig. 3.23. The dimensional accuracy and tensile mechanical properties of TLM alloy tubes with smaller diameters and thinner thicknesses under different heat treatment states are shown in Tables 3.11 and 3.12.

The straightening of metal tubes with common sizes can be realized by traditional methods, such as precision straightener with multiple rolls, flexible straightening, and tension straightening. However, for such TLM alloy tubes with smaller diameters and thinner thicknesses as well as high strength and high elasticity, traditional straightening methods are ineffective and can easily cause brittle fractures. On the basis of considerable research, we used thermal tension straightening for such special tubes with inert gas protection to obtain high straightness of the tubes. Accordingly, we developed the specialized straightening equipment shown in Fig. 3.24 [25].

For metal pipes with small diameters and thin walls, polishing them using mechanical polishing operation is difficult and of low efficiency, while chemical polishing cannot meet the requirements. The reasons

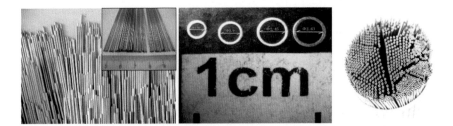

FIGURE 3.23 TLM alloy tubes with smaller diameters and thinner thicknesses.

TABLE 3.11 Dimensional accuracy of typical TLM alloy tubes with small diameter and thinner thickness.

Sample	Parameter	Standard value	Measured value
Φ3 × 0.3 Φ2 × 0.1	Diameter tolerance	± 0.02 mm	3.01 × 0.29, 3.01 × 0.30 mm
	Diameter tolerance	± 0.02 mm	1.99 × 0.10, 2.00 × 0.11 mm
	Surface roughness	≤ 1.6 μm	0.58 μm, 0.60 μm

TABLE 3.12 Mechanical properties of TLM alloy tubes with smaller diameter and thinner thickness after different heat treatments.

Sample	Heat treatment process	R_m (MPa)	R_P (MPa)	E (GPa)	A (%)
Φ3 × 0.2	As-drawn	874	652	61.2	13
	510°C/1 h, AC	838	515	60.8	15
	750°C/1 h, FC	1246	1203	90	10
Φ2 × 0.1	As-drawn	826	702	47.3	3
	510°C/1 h, AC	799	415	66	14
	680°C/1 h, AC + 510°C/4 h, AC	719	612	63	14
	750°C/1 h, FC	1456	–	113.2	–
	750°C/1 h AC + 510°C/4 h, AC	817	724	73	18
Φ2 × 0.18	As-drawn	1050	819	61	3.2
	510°C/1 h, AC	922	808	64.9	17
	750°C/1 h, FC	969	949	66.4	4
Φ1.6 × 0.18	As-drawn	1268	1024	63.2	12
	510°C/1 h, AC	836	–	70.9	10
	750°C/1 h, FC	735	–	60	4

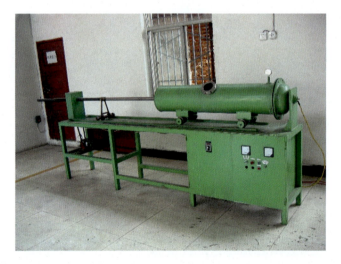

FIGURE 3.24 Straightening equipment of TLM alloy tubes with smaller diameters and thinner thicknesses.

can be summarized as follows. First, owing to the small inner hollow of these pipe (such as Φ3 mm size and smaller), the chemical erosion polishing solution cannot easily interact with the inner surface of the pipe under the influence of surface tension. Second, it is difficult to control the concentration of chemical erosion solution and cleaning time because of the thin walls of such pipes. Third, the dimensional accuracy of the inner wall of the pipe cannot be maintained during polishing. Therefore we independently invented a novel inner surface polishing device (shown in Fig. 3.25), which can effectively solve the polishing problems encountered by TLM Ti alloy pipes with small diameters and thin walls [26].

3.6.2 TLM alloy tubes with thin walls and variable diameters

To meet the needs for special diameters in the field of medical instruments, we first prepared a TLM alloy tube billet with Φ13.8 × 0.3 mm, Φ13.8 × 0.5 mm, Φ15.2 × 0.3 mm, and Φ15.2 × 0.5 mm by a rolling process. Then, by rotary swaging, spinning, and rolling, the large end of the tube is Φ15.2 mm, and the small end is Φ13.8 mm, with a wall thickness of 0.3–0.5 mm (as shown in Fig. 3.26). We have applied for a Chinese invention patent for this process [27,28].

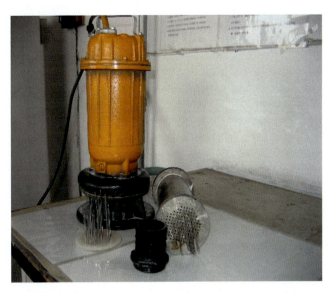

FIGURE 3.25 Novel polishing device for TLM Ti alloy pipes with small diameters and thin walls.

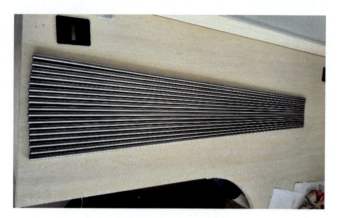

FIGURE 3.26 TLM alloy tubes with variable diameters and thin walls.

3.6.3 TLM alloy wires

Processing of TLM wires can be easily achieved by conventional cold or hot drawing techniques with hot drawing at 700°C–800°C and a deforming rate of single pass controlled at 15% or so, using conventional graphite emulsion as the solid lubricant. With the aid of tube-type furnace heating, the small rods can be drawn into wires with diameters of 1–7 mm, and the hot drawing temperature decreases gradually as the diameter of the wires decreases. To fabricate TLM wires with smaller size and better surface quality, cold drawing at room temperature is further required by means of ordinary commercial lubricating oil.

By studying the tensile mechanical properties of TLM alloy at room temperature and high temperature, we have determined the influence of processing temperature, deformation of cold and hot processing, lubrication, straightening, and heat treatment of finished products on the microstructure and mechanical properties of TLM alloy wires. Finally, we developed TLM alloy wires successfully. The smallest wire can reach 100 μm in diameter, which meets the requirements of medical orthopedic wires, interventional guide wires, surgical sutures, and other devices.

The strength, elastic modulus, and elongation after solid solution treatment of the commonly used Φ1 mm wire are higher than 900 MPa, 60–63 GPa, and 16%–18%, respectively. With further aging treatment, the yield strength and tensile strength can be higher than 1100 and 1200 MPa, respectively, and the elongation rate is about 10%. The relationships between heat treatment and mechanical properties are shown in Fig. 3.27, photos of TLM alloy wires are shown in Fig. 3.28, and the mechanical properties of the wires are listed in Table 3.13.

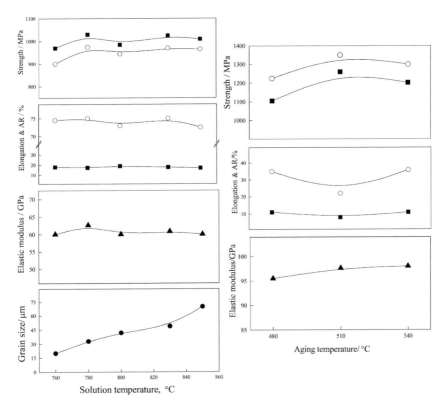

FIGURE 3.27 Relationship between heat treatment and mechanical properties of TLM alloy wires.

3.7 TLM alloy foils

3.7.1 Summary of severe plastic deformation (SPD) processing technology

Recent studies have shown that the elastic modulus of the Ti alloys with superfine crystals or nanocrystals decreases obviously and is closer to that of cortical bone, thus reducing the stress shielding effect caused by the excessive elastic modulus of Ti alloy. Its hardness also increases, which can reduce the formation of articular surface debris [29,30]. This indicates that Ti alloy materials with ultrafine crystals possesses better biomechanical properties than can be found in ordinary Ti alloy materials. Meanwhile, the nanostructures on the surface of Ti alloys provide favorable conditions for the adhesion, differentiation, and proliferation of cells *in vivo*. In addition, the Ti alloys' surface with ultrafine crystals has more grain boundaries, which makes it easy for the surface of the

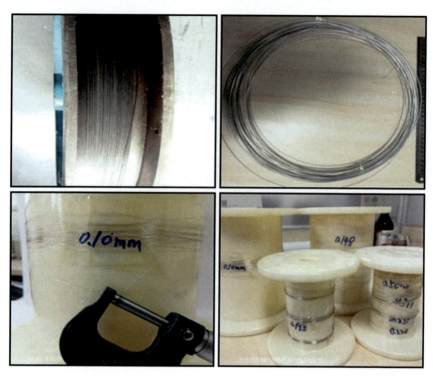

FIGURE 3.28 Photos of TLM alloy wires.

TABLE 3.13 Mechanical properties of typical TLM alloy wires.

Wires	R_m (MPa)	R_p (MPa)	A_5 (%)	E (GPa)	Ra (μm)	Process
Φ6.0	915	866	14	–	–	Hot rolled
Φ4.0	762	300	19	–	–	Hot rolled
Φ3.0	1003	930	16	72	0.81	Cold rolled
Φ2.0	964	861	22	69	2.1	Cold rolled
Φ1.5	981	841	16	73	2.3	Cold rolled
Φ1.0	926	839	15	75	2.82	Cold rolled

material to obtain a large number of free electrons, thus giving the materials higher activation energy and promoting the deposition of bonelike mineral elements, such as calcium and phosphorus, on the surface of the material, accelerating the osseointegration *in vivo* in comparison to the surface with the coarse crystals. Hence the results suggest that Ti alloys with ultrafine crystals on their surface and inside can effectively improve the interface integration of implanted prostheses with bone tissue and are more suitable for use as artificial joint materials [1].

At present, the most advanced techniques for realizing large or SPD, such as high pressure and torsion (HPT), multiple forging, cyclic extrusion-compression, equal channel angular pressing (ECAP), accumulative roll bonding (ARB), repetitive corrugation and straightening, surface mechanical grinding, high-energy ball milling, sandblasting, and shot blasting, can be applied to achieve microscale and nanoscale on the surface and inside of Ti alloys [31]. The mechanical properties of commonly used commercial pure Ti (CP—Ti) materials with coarse grain (TA1—TA4) are tensile strength ≥ 200 MPa, yield strength ≥ 140 MPa, and elongation $\geq 15\%$ [32]. The grain sizes and properties of CP—Ti plates and bars prepared by SPD are compared as shown in Table 3.14, which shows that the strength in ultrafine crystals (basically

TABLE 3.14 Grain size and mechanical properties of CP—Ti bars with ultrafine crystals processed by SPD.

Ti grade	Processing mode and history	Grain size (nm)	R_m (MPa)	A (%)
VT1—0	ECAP	300	810	15
Grade 1	ECAP	400	780	14
Grade 2	Thermomechanical treatment (80%)	70	1150	11
	ECAP + rolling	140	905—937	7—27
	ECAP (10) + CR (77%)	—	945	14.5
	ECAP	—	750	7
	ECAP	300	760	21
	ECAP + CR (70%)	150	1080	32
Grade 3	ECAP + HPT (1.5 GPa)	200	730	25
	ECAP	280	710	14
	ECAP + CR (75%)	100	1150	8
	HPT (5 GPa)	120	950	14
	ECAP (8) + CR (73%) + annealing (300°C, 1 h)	−100	1037	12.5
Grade 4	ECAP + drawing	200—600	1280	10
	ECAP	300	947	25
Grade 2	HPT (3 GPa)	130	940	23

CR, Cold rolling.

in the submicron grade) of CP−Ti far exceeds that of its counterparts with coarse grain.

3.7.2 TLM alloy foil by novel SPD process

The author's research group at NIN in cooperation with the University of Queensland, Australia, has conducted a lot of collaborative research on the preparation of a novel TLM alloy with ultrafine crystals in recent years and has successfully developed an ultrafine-crystalline TLM foil preparation technology with China's intellectual property rights by the ARB technique at room temperature. The average grain size of the TLM alloy prepared under different deforming rates is 80−300 nm, as shown in Fig. 3.29. The tensile strength was increased by 70% deforming to 1220 MPa, the yield stress was doubled to 946 MPa, the plasticity was retained to 4.5%, and the elastic modulus was decreased to less than 40 GPa [33−35]. The increase in strength and grain refinement of the TLM alloy is mainly due to the phase transition (from β-phase to α-phase) that occurs during the deformation process. In addition, preliminary progress has been made in microstructure evolution and thermal stability, and the alloy exhibits obvious equiaxial grains with microscale and nanoscale after annealing treatment. Its microscopic morphologies are shown in Fig. 3.30. The detailed mechanical properties of TLM alloy foils with ultrafine crystals are listed in Table 3.15.

To produce industrial TLM alloy foil with a finer grain, the first step is to obtain thin plates with homogeneous fine grain, which are then successively produced in hot and cold rolling mills with 4, 6, 14, and 20 rollers, in which the foil is cold rolled by a reversible rolling mill with 4 rolls or a

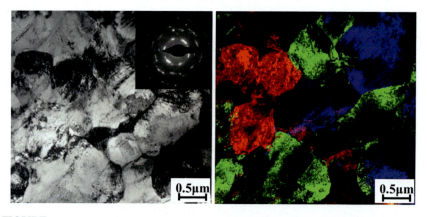

FIGURE 3.29 TEM morphologies of TLM foil with ultrafine crystals prepared by ARB. *Source: data from D. Kent, W.L. Xiao, G. Wang, Z. Yu, M.S. Dargusch. Thermal stability of an ultrafine grain β-Ti alloy, Materials Science & Engineering A 556 (2012) 582−587.*

3.7 TLM alloy foils

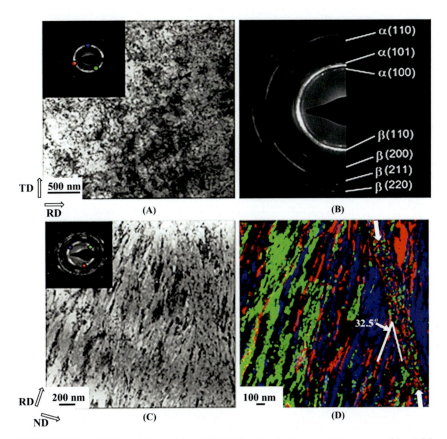

FIGURE 3.30 TEM morphologies of TLM foil with ultrafine crystals prepared by ARB. (A) Bright field image and (B) SADP indexed to the β and α phases from the ND view. (C) Bright field image and (D) composite dark field image from the TD view. *Source: data from D. Kent, G. Wang, Z. Yu, X. Ma, M. Dargusch, Strength enhancement of a biomedical Ti alloy through a modified accumulative roll bonding technique, Journal of the Mechanical Behavior of Biomedical Materials 4 (2011) 405–416.*

TABLE 3.15 Mechanical properties of TLM alloy foil with ultrafine grain by ARB.

Condition	R_p (MPa)	R_m (MPa)	A (%)	E (GPa)	R_p/R_m
1 Layer	445	805	1.5	59.6	0.5528
2 Layers	445	990	3.5	65	0.5
4 Layers	800	1120	4.5	63.7	0.7857
8 Layers	955	1200	5.0	67.4	0.7958

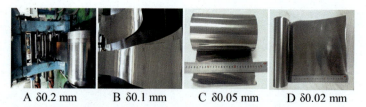

A δ0.2 mm   B δ0.1 mm   C δ0.05 mm   D δ0.02 mm

FIGURE 3.31   TLM alloy foils. (A) δ0.2 mm. (B) δ0.1 mm. (C) δ0.05 mm. (D) δ0.02 mm.

rolling mill with 20 rolls. The production of TLM alloy foils depends mainly on the capacity of the equipment and the intermediate process control. At present, we have successfully produced TLM foils with a minimum thickness of 20 μm and bright and flat surfaces and good quality. The technique has been granted Chinese invention patents [36,37]. Fig. 3.31 shows TLM foil strips with different typical thicknesses.

References

[1] Z. Yu, S. Yu, J. Cheng, X. Ma, Development and application of novel biomedical titanium alloy materials, Acta Metallurgica Sinica 53 (2017) 1238−1264.

[2] Z. Yu, L. Zhou, M. Fan, S. Yuan, Investigation on near-β titanium alloy Ti-5Zr-3Sn-5Mo-15Nb for surgical implant materials, Materials Science Forum 475 (2005) 2353−2358.

[3] Z. Yu, L. Zhou, K. Wang, Research and development of biomedical titanium alloys for surgical implant materials, in: Proc. 7th World Biomaterials Congress, Sydney, 2005.

[4] Z. Yu, L. Zhou, K. Wang, Design and development of biomedical β-type titanium alloy, Rare Metals Letters 35 (2004) 5−10.

[5] Z. Yu, L. Zhou, J. Niu, Q. Huangfu, S. Yuan, β type titanium alloys used in surgical implant materials, Rare Metal Materials and Engineering 35 (2006) 261−265.

[6] Z. Yu, L. Zhou, Influence of martensitic transformation on mechanical compatibility of biomedical β type titanium alloy TLM, Materials Science and Engineering: A 438 (2006) 391−394.

[7] Z. Yu, L. Zhou, X. He, L. Luo, J. Niu, S. Yuan, et al., Development and application of titanium alloy materials for human hard tissue repair and replacement, Functional Materials 37 (2006) 664−669.

[8] Z. Yu, L. Zhou, L. Luo, J. Niu, W. Lixin, S. Yuan, et al., Process, microstructure, properties of newly developed β-type biomedical titanium alloy TLM, Chinese Journal of Rare Metals 30 (2006) 226−230.

[9] Z. Yu, L. Zhou, J. Niu, S. Yuan, X. He, Q. Huangfu, et al., Effect of alloy element, process and heat treatment on mechanical properties of β-type biomedical titanium alloy, Chinese Journal of Rare Metals 31 (2007) 416−419.

[10] Z. Yu, Y. Zhang, J. Niu, J. Han, Q. Huangfu, X. He, et al., Research on heat treatment and material strengthening of near-β titanium alloy Ti4Zr1Sn3Mo25Nb, Rare Metal Materials and Engineering 37 (2007) 542−545.

[11] Z. Yu, G. Wang, X. Ma, M. Dargusch, J. Han, S. Yu, Development of biomedical near β titanium alloys, Materials Science Forum 618 (2009) 303−306.

[12] Z. Yu, Y. Zhang, H. Liu, X. Ma, S. Yu, M. Zhang, Effects of alloy elements, processing and heat treatment on mechanical properties of a near β type biomedical titanium

alloy TiZrMoNb and microstructure analysis, Rare Metal Materials and Engineering 39 (2010) 1795−1801.

[13] X. Ma, Y. Han, Z. Yu, Q. Sun, J. Niu, S. Yuan, Phase transformation and mechanical properties of TLM titanium alloy for orthopaedic implant application, Rare Metal Materials and Engineering 41 (2012) 1535−1538.

[14] Z. Yu, L. Zhou, L. Lijuan, J. Niu, L. Wang, S. Yuan, et al., Investigation on process, microstructure and medical properties of the newly developed near β type biomedical titanium alloy TLM, in: Proc. 11th World Conference on Ti (JIMIC5), 2007, pp. 1425−1428.

[15] T. Jiao, Research on microstucture and mechanical properties of biomedical near β · type TLM Ti alloy thin strip, Northeastern University (2014).

[16] T. Lee, M. Nakai, M. Niinomi, C.H. Park, C.S. Lee, Phase transformation and its effect on mechanical characteristics in warm-deformed Ti-29Nb-13Ta-4.6 Zr alloy, Metals and Materials International 21 (2015) 202−207.

[17] Q. Li, R. Zhang, J. Li, Q. Qi, X. Liu, M. Nakai, et al., Microstructure, mechanical properties, and springback of Ti-Nb alloys modified by Mo addition, Journal of Materials Engineering and Performance 29 (2020) 5366−5373.

[18] W. Zhang, J. Ren, B. Liu, Y. Liu, Z. Wu, J. Qiu, Microstructure and mechanical properties of cold drawn Ti−Nb−Ta−Zr−O wires for orthodontic applications, Metals and Materials International 26 (2020) 973−978.

[19] X. Ma, H. Niu, Z. Yu, S. Yu, C. Wang, Microstructural adjustments and mechanical properties of a cold-rolled biomedical near β − Ti alloy sheet, Rare Metals 37 (2018) 846−851.

[20] C. Jun, J. Liu, Z. Yu, S. Yu, H. Liu, Y. Zhang, One kind of high-strength metastable beta-type Ti alloy bar and its preparation method, Authorization Number: ZL201510184681.6 (2017).

[21] Z. Yu, L. Zhou, J. Deng, H. Gu, Investigation on textures of the alloy Ti-2Al-2.5Zr tube and sheet, Rare Metal Materials and Engineering 29 (2000) 86−89.

[22] Z. Yu, L. Zhou, L. Luo, M. Fan, Y. Fu, Investigation on mechanical compatibility matching for biomedical titanium alloys, Key Engineering Materials 288 (2005) 595−598.

[23] Z. Yu, Y. Lin, W. Wu, D. Li, J. Deng, New lubricating coat for cold drawing of titanium alloy, Rare Metal Materials and Engineering 32 (2003) 205−208.

[24] H. Liu, Z. Yu, Y. Zhang, L. Zhao, W. He, C. Wang, et al., A method for forming small-diameter thin-walled high-strength β titanium alloy pipe, Authorization Number: ZL201510540531.4 (2017).

[25] Z. Yu, J. Niu, Q. Huangfu, S. Liu, X. He, S. Liu, One kind straightening device of small-diameter and thin-walled metal pipe, Authorization Number: ZL200610172259.X (2009).

[26] Z. Yu, J. Niu, Q. Huang, S Yuan, X. He, Y. Zhang, et al., A kind of inner wall surface polishing device of thin-diameter thin-walled metal pipe, Authorization Number: ZL200720147967.8 (2008).

[27] Z. Yu, W. Yun, J. Niu, W. Binbin, C. Wang, Y. Zhang, Rotary forging mechanism and rotary forging processing device for thin-walled, ultra-long, variable-diameter metal bars and pipes, Authorization Number: ZL201510870584.2 (2017).

[28] B. Wen, J. Niu, Z. Yu, W. Yun, Y. Zhang, C. Liu, One kind of spinning device for thin-walled metal pipe, Authorization Number: ZL201520763793.2 (2016).

[29] C.C. Koch, Nanostructured Materials: Processing, Properties and Applications, William Andrew, 2006.

[30] H. Yilmazer, M. Niinomi, M. Nakai, K. Cho, J. Hieda, Y. Todaka, et al., Mechanical properties of a medical β-type titanium alloy with specific microstructural evolution through high-pressure torsion, Materials Science and Engineering: C 33 (2013) 2499−2507.

[31] Z. Yu, M. Xiqun, Y. Sen, Z. Minghua, J. Han, C. Liu, Micro-nano technology and latest progress of biomedical titanium alloy, The Chinese Journal of Nonferrous Metals 20 (2010) 1008–1012.
[32] Z. Yu, S. Yu, M. Zhang, J. Han, X. Ma, Design, development and application of novel biomedical Ti alloy materials applied in surgical implants, Materials China 29 (2010) 35–51.
[33] X. Ma, Z. Yu, J. Niu, S. Yu, C. Liu, Microstructure and properties of ultrafine grained TLM alloy ARB sheet, Rare Metal Materials and Engineering 43 (2014) 152–155.
[34] D. Kent, W. Xiao, G. Wang, Z. Yu, M. Dargusch, Thermal stability of an ultrafine grain β-Ti alloy, Materials Science and Engineering: A 556 (2012) 582–587.
[35] D. Kent, G. Wang, Z. Yu, X. Ma, M. Dargusch, Strength enhancement of a biomedical titanium alloy through a modified accumulative roll bonding technique, Journal of the Mechanical Behavior of Biomedical Materials 4 (2011) 405–416.
[36] X. Ma, Z. Yu, J. Niu, S. Yu, Y. Zhang, C. Liu, et al., One kind method for preparing TLM titanium alloy foil with nanocrystalline structure. Application number: CN 201510219680.0.
[37] X. Ma, Z. Yu, J. Niu, S. Yu, Y. Zhang, S. Liu, et al., One kind method for preparing titanium and titanium alloy foil with ultrafine crystal structure. Application number: CN 201510218340.6.

CHAPTER 4

Biological and mechanical evaluation of TLM alloy

4.1 Biological evaluation of TLM alloy

4.1.1 Biological corrosion behavior

The biological corrosion behavior of Ti3Zr2Sn3Mo25Nb (TLM) alloy was studied in Hank's solution, simulated oral solution (saliva solution), and 0.9% NaCl solution. The pH value of each solution was adjusted to 2.4, 5.4, and 7.4, and then the biological corrosion resistance of TLM alloy was characterized in different solutions [1].

Tables 4.1 and Table 4.2 show the equilibrium potential, corrosion current, cathodic Tafel, and anodic Tafel of TLM alloy processed by two kinds of heat treatment (HT1, HT2) in Hank's solution, NaCl solution, and saliva solution with different pH values. It can be observed that TLM alloy has a broader passivation range in Hank's solution and NaCl solution with different pH values. After being processed by HT2, its passivation current density is smaller, the passivation range and passivation current density are less affected by the pH values of the solution, and the corrosion resistance is better than those of another sample processed by HT1. The passivation range and passivation current density of TLM alloy treated with HT2 are greatly affected by the pH value of the saliva solution.

4.1.2 Hemolysis

To further study the biocompatibility between a novel material and blood, the acute hemolysis of TLM alloy *in vitro* was evaluated by referring to the Pharmaceutical Industry Standard of the People's Republic

TABLE 4.1 Tafel test results of TLM alloy treated with 750°C/1 h, air cooling (AC) (HT1) in different solutions.

Corrosive medium		Equilibrium potential (V)	Cathode Tafel	Anode Tafel	Corrosion current (A cm^{-2})
1750°C/1 h, AC (HT1)	Hanks 2.4	−0.237	4.581	3.714	3.526×10^{-7}
	Hanks 5.4	−0.246	4.646	3.820	5.413×10^{-7}
	Hanks 7.4	−0.292	5.195	3.294	6.858×10^{-8}
	Saliva 2.4	−0.274	5.773	2.904	5.313×10^{-7}
	Saliva 5.4	−0.197	4.707	4.883	5.605×10^{-7}
	Saliva 7.4	−0.244	5.083	3.228	2.557×10^{-7}
	NaCl 2.4	−0.255	4.819	3.373	2.92×10^{-7}
	NaCl 5.4	−0.189	4.842	3.852	1.046×10^{-7}
	NaCl 7.4	−0.247	5.268	3.376	1.241×10^{-7}

TABLE 4.2 Tafel test results of TLM alloy treated with 750°C/1 h, air cooling (AC) + 610°C/1 h, AC (HT2) in different solutions.

Corrosive medium		Equilibrium potential (V)	Cathode Tafel	Anode Tafel	Corrosion current (A cm^{-2})
750°C/1 h, AC + 610°C/1 h, AC (HT2)	Hanks 2.4	−0.328	7.104	3.458	5.340×10^{-8}
	Hanks 5.4	−0.275	4.250	2.653	5.734×10^{-7}
	Hanks 7.4	−0.387	5.584	2.454	1.393×10^{-7}
	Saliva 2.4	−0.181	3.862	3.305	3.465×10^{-7}
	Saliva 5.4	−0.241	4.613	4.056	3.025×10^{-7}
	Saliva 7.4	−0.207	4.915	4.027	1.531×10^{-7}
	NaCl 2.4	−0.432	9.459	2.136	1.145×10^{-7}
	NaCl 5.4	−0.198	4.596	4.097	1.107×10^{-7}
	NaCl 7.4	−0.237	3.888	3.297	3.258×10^{-7}

of China YY/T 0127.1-1993. As a comparison, the hemolysis of dual-phase Ti alloy TC4 (Ti6Al4V), which is commonly used in clinical practice, was also characterized under the same experimental conditions.

1. Materials

   Cylinder samples of TLM alloy and TC4 were selected, the diameter and thickness of which were 4 and 5 mm, respectively. The surface

TABLE 4.3 Absorbance values of Ti alloys.

Materials	TLM	TC4
Absorbance value	0.029	0.027
	0.028	0.023
	0.029	0.026
	0.026	0.024

TABLE 4.4 Hemolysis rates of Ti alloys.

Materials	TLM	TC4
Hemolysis rates	0.697%	0.362%

oxide layer of Ti alloys was removed by grinding, acid washing, ultrasonic cleaning with distilled water for 30 minutes, washing with deionized water 3 times, and drying. A 3-month-old domestic rabbit with a weight of 2.3 kg was selected for the animal experiments.

2. Results

The measured absorbance values of each group are shown in Table 4.3. The hemolysis rate is expressed as a percentage and is calculated according to the following formula (Table 4.4):

$$z = \frac{(D_t - D_{nc})}{(D_{pc} - D_{nc})} \times 100\% \tag{4.1}$$

where Z is the hemolysis rate, D_t is the hemolytic absorbance value of the sample, D_{nc} is the absorbance value of negative contrast, and D_{pc} is the absorbance value of positive contrast.

3. Conclusion

The hemolysis rates of TLM and Ti6Al4V are far less than 5% of the Chinese national standard. They have no acute hemolytic effect and possess good biocompatibility, as shown in Fig. 4.1.

4.1.3 Cytotoxicity

An agar overlay assay method was used in this experiment, and the test method was carried out according to the Pharmaceutical Industry Standard of the People's Republic of China YY/T 0127.9-2001. The

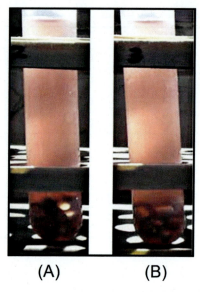

FIGURE 4.1 Hemolysis with anticoagulant-diluted rabbit blood of (A) TLM and (B) Ti6Al4V.

experiment aims to detect the nonspecific cytotoxicity of materials after diffusion through agarose by indirect contact.

1. Materials

    TLM and Ti6Al4V alloys (control sample/group) were used for characterization in this experiment. ATCC CCL1 (NCTC clone 929) [mouse fibroblasts] were thoughtfully selected.

2. Results
    a. The fading index and dissolution index of each sample was calculated as shown in Table 4.5 and Table 4.6.
    b. After deriving the fading index and dissolution index of each test material, we can calculate the average fading index and dissolution index and express the cell reaction according to the formula (4.2). The fading index, dissolution index, and cell reaction of TLM and Ti6Al4V are shown in Table 4.7.

$$\text{Cell reaction} = \frac{\text{Fading index}}{\text{Dissolution index}} \qquad (4.2)$$

3. Conclusion

    The cytotoxicity of the TLM alloy is below grade 1, and there is no obvious cytotoxicity effect, as shown in Fig. 4.2.

TABLE 4.5 Set of fade index.

Fade index	Observation
0	No fading
1	Fading only under the test material
2	The distance of the edge of the fading zone from the edge of the test material (<5.0 mm)
3	The distance of the edge of the fading zone from the edge of the test material (5.0–10.0 mm)
4	The distance of the edge of the fading zone from the edge of the test material (>10.0 mm)
5	All fading

TABLE 4.6 Set of dissolution index.

Dissolution index	Observation
0	No cytolysis occurred
1	Cytolysis <20%
2	Cytolysis between 20% and 40%
3	Cytolysis between 40% and 60%
4	Cytolysis between 60% and 80%
5	Cytolysis more than 80%

4.1.4 Genotoxicity

The genotoxicity of the related materials was tested by the *Salmonella typhimurium* reverse mutation assay (Ames test). The plate incorporation method refers to the relevant parts of Medical Industry Standard of the People's Republic of China YY/T 0127.10-2001, and Technical Standards for Health Food Inspection and Evaluation composed by the Ministry of Health of the People's Republic of China. Four strains of histidine-deficient *S. typhimurium* were chosen in the experiment in TA97, TA98, TA100, and TA102.

1. Results

    The number of recurrent colonies in each dose group and the control group was named $\bar{x} \pm S$. The results of TLM alloy are shown in Table 4.8 and Table 4.9.

TABLE 4.7 Fade index and dissolution index.

Materials	Fade index	Dissolution index	Cellular reaction
TLM	1	0	0/1
	0	0	
	0	0	
	0	0	
	0	0	
	0	0	
TC4	1	0	0/0
	0	0	
	0	0	
	0	0	
	0	0	
	0	0	

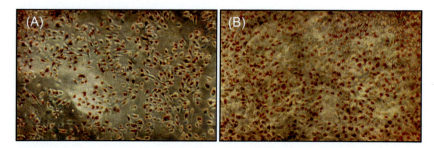

FIGURE 4.2 Cytotoxicity of (A) TLM and (B) Ti6Al4V by agar overlay test.

2. Conclusion

The number of recurrent bacterial colonies of TLM in each dose group was not more than twice the number of natural ones. The results of the Ames test were negative. No point mutagenesis was found in the TLM alloy within the range of 0.16–100 μL/vessel [2], as shown in Fig. 4.3.

4.1.5 Chronic toxicity

The chronic toxicity test of TLM and TC4 (Ti6Al4V) alloy refers to the GB/T 16886.1–2003 evaluation and experiment and *Supervision and*

TABLE 4.8 Ames statistical results of TLM alloy.

Strain	TA97		TA98		TA100		TA102	
Group	S−9 (−)	S−9 (+)	S−9 (−)	S−9 (+)	S−9 (−)	S−9 (+)	S−9 (−)	S−9 (+)
Natural recurrent	154 ± 13	153 ± 20	39 ± 4	40 ± 4	189 ± 13	178 ± 16	288 ± 37	290 ± 18
100 μL/vessel	147 ± 12	144 ± 21	36 ± 6	38 ± 2	187 ± 12	181 ± 32	301 ± 20	284 ± 22
20 μL/vessel	143 ± 22	145 ± 16	38 ± 4	36 ± 6	159 ± 23	185 ± 16	301 ± 16	297 ± 13
4 μL/vessel	152 ± 28	149 ± 18	38 ± 4	38 ± 6	158 ± 28	173 ± 28	279 ± 27	294 ± 27
0.8 μL/vessel	140 ± 16	147 ± 12	37 ± 7	35 ± 2	174 ± 9	175 ± 26	281 ± 11	283 ± 8
0.16 μL/vessel	137 ± 25	138 ± 20	33 ± 2	36 ± 4	163 ± 16	160 ± 28	289 ± 25	295 ± 26

Number of recurrent bacterial colonies ($\bar{x} \pm S$) (first time).

TABLE 4.9 Ames statistical results of TLM alloy.

Strain	TA97		TA98		TA100		TA102	
Group	S–9 (–)	S–9 (+)	S–9 (–)	S–9 (+)	S–9 (–)	S–9 (+)	S–9 (–)	S–9 (+)
Natural recurrent	139 ± 19	139 ± 14	37 ± 5	36 ± 2	194 ± 9	184 ± 8	296 ± 12	293 ± 20
100 μL/vessel	141 ± 20	139 ± 25	36 ± 4	37 ± 6	185 ± 23	181 ± 13	281 ± 20	284 ± 14
20 μL/vessel	143 ± 11	149 ± 6	37 ± 6	39 ± 3	181 ± 17	181 ± 12	285 ± 14	284 ± 8
4 μL/vessel	147 ± 14	158 ± 13	35 ± 4	39 ± 6	182 ± 15	193 ± 8	283 ± 23	286 ± 12
0.8 μL/vessel	146 ± 9	145 ± 21	35 ± 5	38 ± 4	173 ± 16	199 ± 12	286 ± 13	297 ± 12
0.16 μL/vessel	145 ± 23	133 ± 22	37 ± 6	42 ± 10	185 ± 11	181 ± 17	293 ± 8	279 ± 15

Number of recurrent bacterial colonies ($\bar{x} \pm S$) (second time).

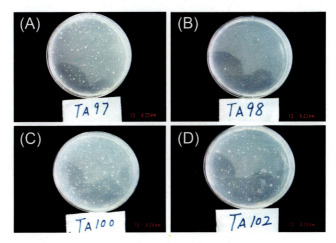

FIGURE 4.3 Genetic toxicity test of histidine-deficient *Salmonella typhimurium* effected by TLM leach liquor. (A) TA97. (B) TA98. (C) TA100. (D) TA102.

Management and Evaluation of Medical Devices [M] (China Medical Science and Technology Press). All experimental animals were sprague dawley (SD) rats. According to the general toxicity observation index after animal exposure, the animals from the new TLM alloy groups and TC4 control groups were all in normal degree, and no signs of poisoning were shown, as seen in Tables 4.10 and 4.11. Statistical results showed that there were no significant differences in the five indicators of weight gain, liver, spleen, kidney, and brain organ index of male rats ($P > .05$).

The results of hematology showed that there was a significant difference in the BUN index in male rats ($P < 0.05$). The datum of TC4 is higher than that of TLM. There were no significant differences in white cell count (WBC), red cell count (RBC), hemoglobin (HGB), hematocrit (HCT), alanine aminotransferase (ALT), aspartate aminotransferase (AST), total protein (TP), and blood urea nitrogen (BUN) ($P > .05$) for TC4 and TLM, as shown in Table 4.12.

The statistical results for female rats showed that there were no significant differences in RBC, WBC, HGB, HCT, BUN, AST, ALT, and TP ($P > .05$) for TC4 and TLM, as shown in Table 4.13.

Among all hematological indexes, the BUN value of male rats in the TC4 group was higher than that in the TLM group ($P < .05$). The following reasons were considered: (1) renal toxicity caused by the toxicity of the alloy impairing the kidney function of male rats and (2) unknown interference factors.

After the new TLM alloy was implanted into the thigh muscle of SD rats, no obvious abnormalities or evidence of toxicity was found during the observation period compared with TC4 alloy, as shown in Fig. 4.4.

TABLE 4.10 Weight gain and other organ index of male SD rats. SD, Sprague dawley.

Materials	Weight gain	Liver	Spleen	Kidney	Brain
TC4	87.564 ± 1.3967	4.087 ± 5.801 × 10^{-2}	0.407 ± 1.588 × 10^{-2}	0.744 ± 1.637 × 10^{-2}	0.286 ± 3.553 × 10^{-3}
TLM	87.196 ± 1.5654	4.018 ± 8.883 × 10^{-2}	0.423 ± 1.606 × 10^{-2}	0.760 ± 1.894 × 10^{-2}	0.291 ± 4.216 × 10^{-3}

TABLE 4.11 Weight gain and other organ index of female SD rats.

Materials	Weight gain	Liver	Spleen	Kidney	Brain
TC4	84.1 ± 1.3956	$4.08 \pm 5.902 \times 10^{-2}$	$0.42 \pm 1.237 \times 10^{-2}$	$0.73 \pm 2.063 \times 10^{-2}$	0.29 ± 1.1485
TLM	81.5 ± 1.3729	$4.06 \pm 5.921 \times 10^{-2}$	$0.41 \pm 1.617 \times 10^{-2}$	$0.760 \pm 1.568 \times 10^{-2}$	$0.29 \pm 4.000 \times 10^{-3}$

TABLE 4.12 Test results of the hematological index in male rats. WBC, White cell count; RBC, red cell count; HGB, hemoglobin; HCT, hematocrit; ALT: alanine aminotransferase; AST, aspartate aminotransferase; TP, total protein; BUN, blood urea nitrogen.

Materials	WBC	RBC	HGB	HCT
TC4	7.084 ± 0.4154	8.5484 ± 0.1261	148.52 ± 1.1946	0.485 ± 6.033 × 10^{-3}
TLM	6.96 ± 0.4907	8.97 ± 0.1962	151.64 ± 2.0896	0.5075 ± 9.182 × 10^{-3}

Materials	ALT	AST	TP	BUN
TC4	88.96 ± 2.5829	149.92 ± 4.7413	75.0 ± 0.4055	7.984 ± 0.1428
TLM	95.76 ± 3.2328	178.4 ± 11.7869	77.912 ± 1.44	6.248 ± 0.1851

TABLE 4.13 Test results of the hematological index in female rats. WBC, White cell count; RBC, red cell count; HGB, hemoglobin; HCT, hematocrit; ALT: alanine aminotransferase; AST, aspartate aminotransferase; TP, total protein; BUN, blood urea nitrogen.

Materials	WBC	RBC	HGB	HCT
TC4	6.748 ± 0.6334	7.6492 ± 0.1424	136.76 ± 1.8835	0.45652 ± 6.6005 × 10^{-3}
TLM	8.02 ± 0.3638	7.8612 ± 0.02382	141.4 ± 0.8981	0.46252 ± 1.6724 × 10^{-3}

Materials	ALT	AST	TP	BUN
TC4	78.92 ± 4.1705	172.88 ± 12.7213	71.76 ± 1.4998	8.38 ± 0.2274
TLM	81.44 ± 4.0113	152.6 ± 7.9143	72.344 ± 0.9898	7.676 ± 0.2193

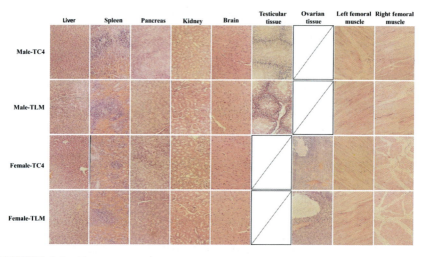

FIGURE 4.4 Chronic toxicity evaluation of TLM alloy.

4.1.6 Skin sensitization and irritation

In this study, skin sensitization and irritation of TLM and TC4 (control group) alloy were studied by the maximum dose method according to the ISO 10993-10:1995 standard. The results are shown in Table 4.14. The degree of erythema and edema response of the applied positions in each group was evaluated according to the scoring standards specified in Table 4.15.

Animals in each group were normally active and fed normally. The dressings were well fixed to ensure nondisplacement of the dressings. The evaluation results of each group according to the skin reaction classification system in Table 4.15 are shown in Table 4.16. The primary stimulation index (PII) of each material is shown in Table 4.17. The results show that TLM and Ti6Al4V have no skin sensitization and very slight irritation, as shown in Figs. 4.5 and 4.6.

4.1.7 Oral irritation

According to the ISO 10993-10:1995 standard for oral irritation test, golden hamsters aged 60–70 days were selected for the experiment of TLM and TC4 (control group). The animal's erythema reaction scores according to the oral response classification system are given in Table 4.18.

After observation for 2 weeks, all animals showed normal activities, normal diet, and no systemic adverse reactions. According to the

TABLE 4.14 Concentration in different stage for materials (%).

Materials	Intradermal induced		Local induced		Local stimulated	
	Rabbit quantity	Concentration	Rabbit quantity	Concentration	Rabbit quantity	Concentration
TLM	3	100	4	100	4	100
TC4	3	100	4	100	4	100

TABLE 4.15 Classification and degree for skin reactions.

Generate erythema and eschar	Score	Generate edema	Score
No erythema	0	No edema	0
Slight erythema	1	Slight edema	1
Obvious erythema	2	Obvious edema	2
Moderate erythema	3	Moderate edema	3
Severe erythema and slight eschar	4	Severe edema	4

TABLE 4.16 Sensitization rate and reaction scores of two types of Ti alloys.

Materials	Numbers of animals	Numbers of sensitizations	Sensitization rate	Erythema score	Edema score	Skin reaction score
TLM	15	0	0	0	0	0
TC4	15	0	0	0	0	0

TABLE 4.17 Primary stimulation index (PII) of two types of Ti alloy.

	TLM	TC4
PII	0	0
Reaction type	Very slightly	Very slightly

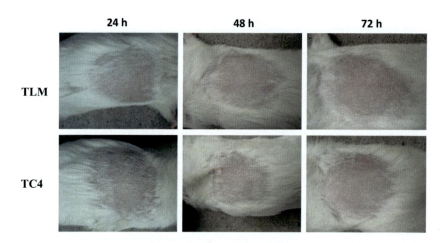

FIGURE 4.5 Test of skin sensitization of TLM and TC4 alloys.

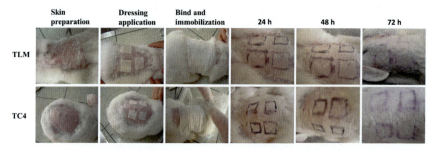

FIGURE 4.6 Test of skin irritation of TLM and TC4 alloy.

TABLE 4.18 Classification for oral reactions.

Generate erythema and eschar	Score
No erythema	0
Slight erythema	1
Obvious erythema	2
Moderate erythema	3
Severe erythema and slightly eschar	4

TABLE 4.19 Oral reaction scores for TLM and Ti6Al4V.

Materials	Quantity	Score for sample	Average score
TLM	10	0	0
TC4	10	0	0

TABLE 4.20 Histological evaluation scores.

Materials	Quantity	Score for sample	Score for blanks	Stimulation index	Extent of reaction
TLM	10	0	0	0	No
TC4	10	0	0	0	No

classification system in Table 4.18, the scoring results of the erythema reaction of each group of animals are shown in Table 4.19.

The tissue sections of the TLM group showed that the epithelial continuity was intact. As depicted in Table 4.20 and Fig. 4.7, no cell deformation or flattening and no ulcers or erosions were found. The cell layers were clear and evenly arranged. No leukocyte infiltration in the connective tissue, no vascular congestion, and no tissue edema were found. These results show that both Ti alloys have no oral irritation [3].

4.1.8 Intradermal reaction

According to ISO 10993-10:1995 and ISO/TR7406, the intradermal reaction of TLM and TC4 (control group) were tested. Healthy young albino rabbits in the same strain with weight between 2.1 and 2.5 kg, were selected, with six rabbits per group.

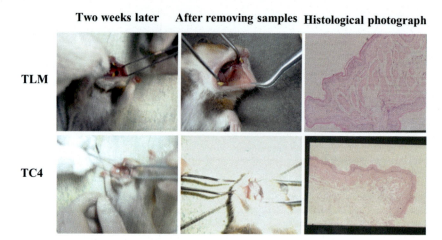

FIGURE 4.7 Oral mucosal irritation test of TLM and TC4 alloy.

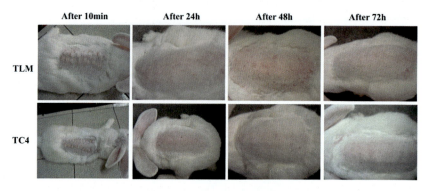

FIGURE 4.8 Intradermal reaction test of TLM and TC4 alloy.

The results are depicted in Fig. 4.8, and the scores are listed in Table 4.21. The primary irritation indexes of TLM and TC4 were both 0, and the type of rabbit intradermal irritation was very mild. From the perspective of intradermal reaction, both materials have good biosafety, as shown in Table 4.22.

4.1.9 Subcutaneous, muscle, and bone implantation

1. Test of subcutaneous and muscle implantation
    According to the GB/T16886.6-1997 standard, the test pieces used in the experiment were all processed into cylindrical rods with a diameter of 1.0 mm and a length of 10.0 mm. The experimental design was divided into two groups: test piece 1 and test piece 2 for

4.1 Biological evaluation of TLM alloy

TABLE 4.21 Classification for intradermal reaction.

Reaction	Score
Generate erythema and eschar	
No erythema	0
Slight erythema	1
Obvious erythema	2
Moderate erythema	3
Severe erythema and slight eschar	4
Generate edema	
No edema	0
Slightly edema	1
Obvious edema	2
Moderate edema ($\sim$1 mm)	3
severe edema ($>$1 mm)	4
highest scores	8

TABLE 4.22 Primary stimulation index (PII) for intradermal reaction.

	TLM	TC4
PII	0.0	0.0
Reaction type	Very slightly	Very slightly

TLM, control material for TC4. Thirty healthy adult house mice, male and female, with a weight of 1.6 ± 0.6 kg were selected. The mice were divided into a subcutaneous implantation group and a muscle implantation group, with 15 animals in each group.

There were no significant differences in the test results between the TLM specimen and the TC4 specimen at different periods. Both Ti alloys meet the standard and show excellent biocompatibility. As is shown in Fig. 4.9, the surface of the TLM alloy exhibited a brushlike tearing phenomenon, which became more obvious with time, indicating soft tissue adhesion on the material surface. This phenomenon provides a basis to eliminate the potential gap between the surgical implant material and the soft tissue [4,5].

2. Bone implantation test

This test refers to the GB/T 16886.6−2001. All samples of TLM and TC4 alloys were made into cylinders with a diameter of 2 mm and a

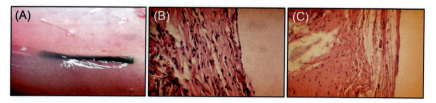

FIGURE 4.9 Test of muscle implantation of TLM (A) in 12 weeks, (B) in 6 weeks (10 × 40 Hematoxylin and eosin (HE) staining), and (C) in 12 weeks (10 × 20 HE).

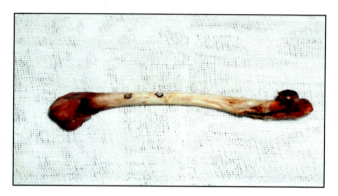

FIGURE 4.10 The positions of the implanted TLM and Ti6Al4V.

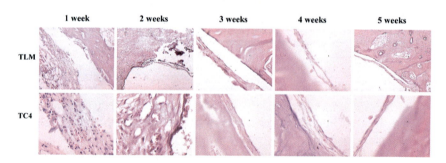

FIGURE 4.11 The microanatomy around the implanted TLM and Ti6Al4V alloy.

length of 6 mm, which were sterilized at high temperature for use. The experimental animals were healthy Chinese rabbits, half male and half female, weighing about 2 kg.

Within 3 days after the operation, the rabbit had a regular diet, the wound healed well, there was no obvious exudation, and there were no adhesion, hyperemia, edema, necrosis, or other abnormalities between the implants and the surrounding tissues. During each observation period, no obvious osteolysis, bone resorption, abnormal bone hyperplasia, or other

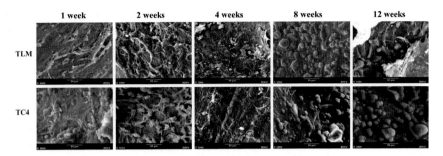

FIGURE 4.12 The microanatomy around the implanted TLM and TC4 alloy.

phenomena were found around the TLM and TC4 control samples. There were no significant differences in the test results between the two materials [6,7]. The results are shown in Figs. 4.10−4.12.

4.2 Biomechanical compatibility of TLM alloy

4.2.1 Conception of biomechanical compatibility

Among medical metal materials, Ti and its alloys are generally recognized as biocompatible materials. However, biomedical materials, especially those used in surgical implantation and orthopedic surgery, require not only good biocompatibility, but also good biomechanical compatibility; that is, their elasticity and allowable strain must match the natural bone so as to avoid stress shielding, which may induce implant failure.

In this chapter, the author summarizes the relationship between biomedical metal materials and mechanics of the body and proposed the concept of biomechanical compatibility, which implies that the implant materials should have sufficient strength to transfer uniform load continuously and everlastingly to the bone and that there is a good match between the donor and the recipient at the binding interface [8]. Biomechanical compatibility evaluation involves the mechanical properties of materials, including strength, plasticity, elastic modulus, wear resistance, fatigue performance, and superelasticity. It is a concept of comprehensive evaluation. If the comprehensive mechanical properties of these materials are reflected in different implants, they should have reliability, stability, durability, and adaptability of bonelike function. Therefore it is not easy to judge the biomechanical compatibility of biomaterials simply by getting the low elastic modulus close to or matching that of human bone tissue.

We believe that medical metal materials must have sufficient strength and toughness to ensure their effectiveness and reliability after implantation. But the pursuit of static mechanical properties, such as high strength, low elastic modulus, and high plastic toughness, is far from the actual situation of human bone tissue. More in-depth study of dynamic mechanical properties is needed. In other words, to ensure the long-term harmonious coexistence of Ti joints, dental implants, and the like and bone under the dynamic and static conditions of the human body, it is also necessary to study the biomechanical properties, biotribological behavior, and micromechanics of implant material and its surface and interface under long-term movement and complex stress conditions in the *in vivo* physiological environment.

Therefore research on biomedical metal materials with excellent biocompatibility and biomechanical compatibility and exploration of the relationship between their composition, microstructure, mechanical properties, and biological properties should be the everlasting goal and direction pursued by biomaterials scientists.

4.2.2 Phase transformation and biomechanical match of TLM alloy

According to the phase transformation temperature of TLM alloy and the experience of heat treatment process of β-type Ti alloy, we have developed a new heat treatment system for medical TLM alloy, as shown in Table 4.23. The solid solution and aging heat treatment experiments of semifinished products were carried out in an ordinary resistance furnace and in atmosphere, respectively. The heat treatment of finished products was carried out in ordinary resistance furnace, argon protection state, or vacuum furnace. Table 4.24 shows the typical mechanical properties of hot rolled TLM bar, showing excellent processing plasticity and deformation ability.

TABLE 4.23 Designing scheme of heat treating for TLM alloy.

	Processing	Solution treatment	Aging treatment
TLM	Φ12 mm/hot rolled in β phase region (RP1) Φ8 mm/ hot rolled in α + β phase region (RP2)	1. (800–830°C)/1–2 h/WQ or AC (ST1) 2. (730–760°C)/1–2 h/WQ or AC (ST2) 3. (660–690°C)/1–2 h/WQ or AC (ST3)	1. 510°C/4–12 h/AC (A1) 2. 560°C/4–12 h/AC (A2) 3. 610°C/4–12 h/AC (A3)

AC, Air cooling; *WQ*, water quenching.

4.2 Biomechanical compatibility of TLM alloy

TABLE 4.24 Mechanical property of TLM rods.

R_m (MPa)	R_p (MPa)	A (%)	Z (%)	E (GPa)	Notes
790/775	390/435	15/21	56	58/76	Φ12 mm rod by hot rolling in β phase region from 5-kg ingot
965/1020	825/900	13/13	—	77/83	Φ8 mm rod by hot rolling in α + β phase region from 5-kg ingot
690	340	19	81	55	Φ8 mm rod by hot rolling in β phase region from 25-kg ingot
815/830	430/455	17/22	83/86	53/52	Φ8 mm rod by hot rolling in α + β phase region from 25-kg ingot

TABLE 4.25 Effect of metastable phases on the mechanical property of TLM alloy.

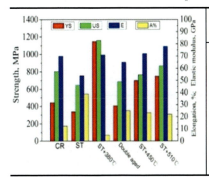

Microstructure evolution	E (GPa)	R_m (MPa)	A (%)
β + α″	54	645	39
β + partial α″ + mass ω (few nanometers)	48	1270	6
β + partial α″ + mass ω (some 10 nanometers)	62	1160	13
β + α″ + α	75	765	23
β + α	78	868	22

The mechanical properties of TLM alloy are closely related to its complex phase transition microstructure, as shown in Table 4.25. The TLM alloy phase transition process can be controlled by controlling the processing, solid solution, and aging parameters. The growth rule and decomposition mechanism of substable phase in the TLM alloy are further analyzed [9,10], as shown in Fig. 4.13.

In fact, by comparing the mechanical properties of cortical bone with that of commonly used implant materials, such as Ti6Al4V, CP–Ti, 316L stainless steel, CoCrMo alloy, and novel TLM alloy, it can be found that TLM alloy with high strength and low modulus has the comprehensive mechanical properties most similar to those of body bone, as shown in Table 4.26. This enables it to avoid the occurrence of stress shielding to the greatest possible extent.

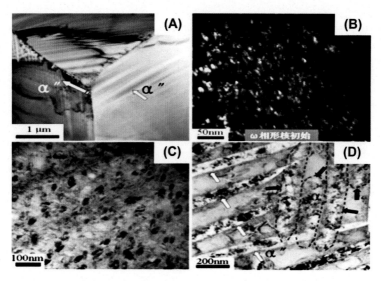

FIGURE 4.13 TEM images of phase transformation from β to α in TLM alloy: (A) A volume fraction of parallel α″ formation after solution treatment and water quenching. (B) Dark field morphology of initial metastable ω phase. (C) Bright field morphology of grown metastable ω phase and (D) α martensite formation from β matrix.

TABLE 4.26 Mechanical property comparison between bone and biometals.

Materials	R_m (MPa)	E (GPa)	R_m/ρ (MPa/g cm^{-3})	R_p/R_m (%)	R_p/E (%)
Cortical bone	30–200	15–26	166	High	0.67
TLM	800–1200	60–90	235	High	0.90
Ti6Al4V	900–1200	110	266	High	0.85
CP–Ti	200–500	105–110	111	High	0.66
316L	465–950	170–200	120	Proper	
CoCrMo	860–1250	240–270	137	Proper	

4.2.3 Grain refinement and the match of strength and toughness of TLM alloy

The novel TLM alloy is a near β-type Ti alloy, which generally presents an equiaxial structure that is mainly composed of a substable phase and a small amount of primary α phase under the state of solid solution treatment. The alloy possesses lower strength and higher elongation, which is convenient for material processing at this state. After the solid solution and aging treatment, the substable β phase is transformed into a small secondary α phase; the strength and elastic modulus are thereby increased for the dispersion and finer-grain effect of these second α phase, while the elongation and fracture toughness are decreased. So selecting the proper heat treatment system to control the appropriate grain size and volume fraction of the α precipitated phase to adjust comprehensive mechanical properties of materials can enable the materials meet different practical requirements [8].

To further improve the quality of Ti alloy materials, the grain refining technology of TLM alloy was realized based on the idea of micro-nano and homogenization [11,12]. By using multipasses, large deformation of cold rolling provided large strain, and the grain structure of TLM alloy is fully refined (according to the continuous dynamic recrystallization mechanism). Combining the multirolling with the short-term annealing process (aiming at eliminating the work hardening and maximally improving the finer-grain strengthening effect), TLM alloy foil can reach a high strength (1000 MPa) and low modulus (50 GPa) with good plastic toughness (10%). The microstructure of TLM alloy foil is shown in Fig. 4.14.

4.2.4 Superelasticity of TLM alloy

The novel near β-Ti TLM alloy exhibits superelastic properties, and its microscopic mechanism is different from that of the traditional TiNi alloy with memory and superelasticity (intermetallic compound).

1. The effect of tensile deformation temperature on superelasticity
   When the tensile deformation of the hot rolled TLM is at 3%, the cyclic loading and unloading curves at different temperatures are as shown in Fig. 4.15. At room temperature, after it has been stretched to 3% and cycle loaded and unloaded five times, the loading and unloading curves overlap. But while the tensile loading and unloading cycles of the same strain are performed at 150°C and 330°C, the maximum stress decreases and the residual strain increases with the increases in cycle.
2. The effect of tensile deformation on superelasticity of TLM

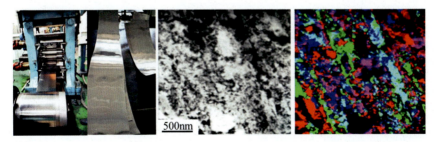

FIGURE 4.14 TLM foil and its microstructure produced by severe plastic deformation.

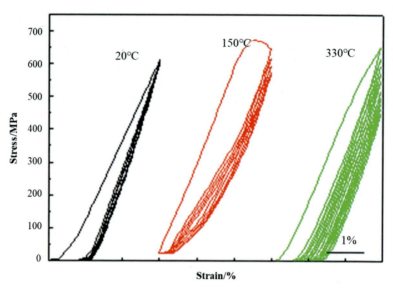

FIGURE 4.15 Loading-unloading curves of hot rolled TLM alloy in 3% at different temperature. Source: *data from Z. Yu, Y. Zheng, J. Niu, Q. Huangfu, Y. Zhang, S. Yu, Microstructure and wear resistance of Ti-3Zr-2Sn-3Mo-15Nb (TLM) alloy, Transactions of Nonferrous Metals Society of China 17 (2007) 495s–499s.*

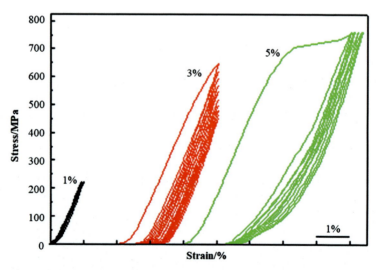

FIGURE 4.16 Loading-unloading curves of hot rolled TLM alloy with different strains at 330°C. Source: *data from Z. Yu, Y. Zheng, J. Niu, Q. Huangfu, Y. Zhang, S. Yu, Microstructure and wear resistance of Ti-3Zr-2Sn-3Mo-15Nb (TLM) alloy, Transactions of Nonferrous Metals Society of China 17 (2007) 495s–499s.*

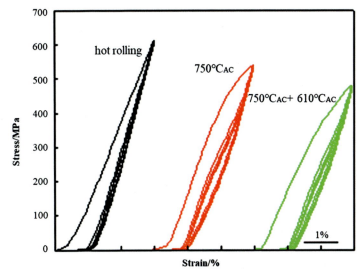

FIGURE 4.17 Loading-unloading curves of TLM alloy with different heat treatments.

Fig. 4.16 shows the loading and unloading curves with different strains (1%, 3%, 5%) at 330°C of the hot rolled TLM. It can be observed that the elastic strain increases a lot with the increase of deformation.

3. The effect of different treatment processes on superelasticity

Fig. 4.17 shows the curves of 3% strain loading and unloading of TLM after three treatments with hot rolling, 750°C/air cooling (AC) and 750°C/AC + 610°C/AC. After cyclic loading and unloading five times, the recoverable elastic strains are not much different.

4.2.5 Shape memory capability of TLM alloy

The shape memory effect of TLM alloy was evaluated by the bending test, including the influence of cyclic deformation on the phase transformation temperature and the influence of bending deformation temperature, bending deformation amount, and cyclic deformation times on the shape memory effect of TLM alloy. The different states of TLM were unloaded after 4.9% bending deformation at different temperatures (−70°C, −40°C, −10°C, RT, 37°C, 70°C) and heated to above M_f temperature, and then the shape recovery rate was measured. As shown in Fig. 4.18 and Table 4.27, the shape recovery rates of the alloy processed with 680°C/AC, 680°C/water quenching (WQ), 750°C/AC, 820°C/AC, and 820°C/WQ does not change much with the increase in bending deformation temperature. With the increase in bending deformation temperature, the shape recovery rate of hot rolled TLM gradually

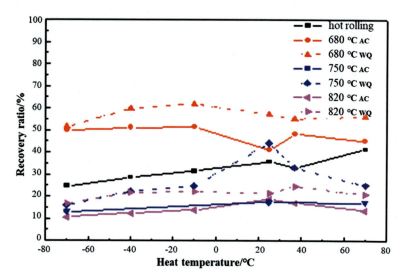

FIGURE 4.18 Effect of bending deformation temperature on the shape recovery rate of TLM alloy. *Source: data from Z. Yu, Y. Zheng, J. Niu, Q. Huangfu, Y. Zhang, S. Yu, Microstructure and wear resistance of Ti-3Zr-2Sn-3Mo-15Nb (TLM) alloy, Transactions of Nonferrous Metals Society of China 17 (2007) 495s–499s.*

TABLE 4.27 Start and final reverse transformation temperature of martensite of TLM by different processes.

	Hot rolled	680°C/AC	680°C/WQ	750°C/WQ
M_s (°C)	140	145	160	161
M_s (°C) (15 cycles)	117	135	93	161
M_f (°C)	325	250	248	257
M_f (°C) (1 cycle)	171	182	200	197

AC, Air cooling; WQ, water quenching.
Source: *data from Z. Yu, Y. Zheng, L. Zhou, B. Wang, J. Niu, H. Qiang, et al., Shape memory effect and superelastic property of a novel Ti-3Zr-2Sn-3Mo-15Nb alloy, Rare Metal Materials and Engineering 37 (2008) 1–5.*

increases. The TLM with hot rolled, 680°C/AC, 680°C/WQ, and 750°C/WQ have higher recovery rates.

Fig. 4.19A shows the effect of different bending deformations (1.8%, 2.4%, 4.9%, 6.7%, 9.3%, 11.5% at room temperature) on the shape memory effect of different processed TLM. Fig. 4.19B shows the effect of different bending deformations on the shape memory effect of it after 10 cycles of bending deformation. As the bending deformation increases, the shape recovery rate of TLM decreases. When the bending

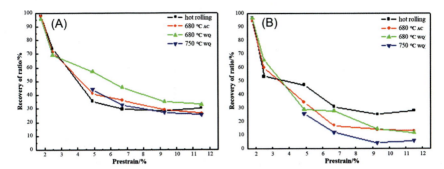

FIGURE 4.19 Effect of bending and cycle deformation on the shape recovery rate of different processed TLM. (A) Noncycle. (B) After 10 cycles. Source: *data from Z. Yu, Y. Zheng, J. Niu, Q. Huangfu, Y. Zhang, S. Yu, Microstructure and wear resistance of Ti-3Zr-2Sn-3Mo-15Nb (TLM) alloy, Transactions of Nonferrous Metals Society of China 17 (2007) 495s—499s.*

deformation is 1.8%, TLM processed with hot rolling, 680°C/AC, and 680°C/WQ is almost completely restored after heating. This is because the increase in deformation results in irreversible plastic deformation. As the bending deformation increases, the proportion of plastic deformation increases, and the shape recovery rate of the sample decreases rapidly. After 10 cycles of bending deformation, the process for the stable shape recovery rate is as follows: hot rolled state > 680°C/AC ≈ 680°C/WQ > 750°C/WQ.

In summary, TLM processed with hot rolling, 680°C/AC, 680°C/WQ, and 750°C/WQ have higher shape recovery rates. The maximum bending recovery strain is less than 3%. This provides useful information for applications involving surgical implants in soft tissue, such as intravascular stents [13—19].

4.2.6 High-cycle fatigue deforming performance of TLM alloy

High-cycle fatigue performance refers to the maximum stress that does not cause a break under repeated or alternating stress and characterizes the ability of a material to withstand repeated loads. After 10^7 cycles, the fatigue strength of the TLM exceeds 510 MPa. The S—N curve is shown in Fig. 4.20. The fatigue limits of the TC4 measured at the same conditions is 350 MPa [1].

As was stated earlier in the chapter, the biomedical near-β Ti alloy TLM has excellent characteristics such as high strength, low elastic modulus, and high fatigue limit, which can allow the novel alloy not only to be applied in the orthopedic and interventional fields, such as artificial joints, spinal internal fixation systems, dental implants, and

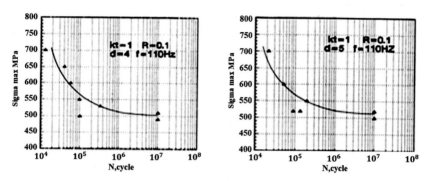

FIGURE 4.20 Fatigue property curves of hot rolled TLM bar (Φ16 mm).

vascular stents, but also to be used in other military and civilian fields, such as acting as high-strength fasteners (e.g., rivets, bolts), elastic components, and bulletproof or impact-resistant parts.

4.2.7 Low-cycle fatigue deforming performance of TLM alloy

The low-cycle fatigue deformation value is lower, usually less than 10^5, and the high-cycle fatigue value is higher, usually more than 10^5. Generally, the lower stress within the elasticity occurs for high-cycle fatigue deformation, while relatively high and plastic deformation often occurs for low-cycle fatigue deformation. The research on low-cycle fatigue deformation of Ti and its alloys is less than that of other metal materials, and the research data on biomedical Ti alloys are even lower. Owing to the high stress level of materials undergoing low-cycle fatigue, the low-cycle fatigue deforming test of biomedical Ti alloy can evaluate the properties of materials under high stress levels and also estimate the fatigue fracture life of materials, thus providing a technical reference for designing artificial joints, dental implants, and other products of Ti alloys.

The low-cycle fatigue properties of TLM alloy in the solid solution state and the aging state were compared, and it was found that the elastic modulus of the former gradually increased during the fatigue deformation process, while the elastic modulus of the latter remained unchanged, as shown in Fig. 4.21.

Fatigue life is the evaluation of the performance of the material and an important index in the material selection. The fatigue life of low-cycle fatigue is expressed with the strain-life relationship, in which the elastic strain amplitude is $\Delta\varepsilon_e/2$, the plastic strain amplitude is $\Delta\varepsilon_p/2$,

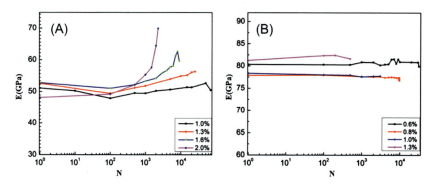

FIGURE 4.21 Variation of elastic modulus of TLM with different fatigues cycles. (A) Solid solutioned. (B) Aging annealed.

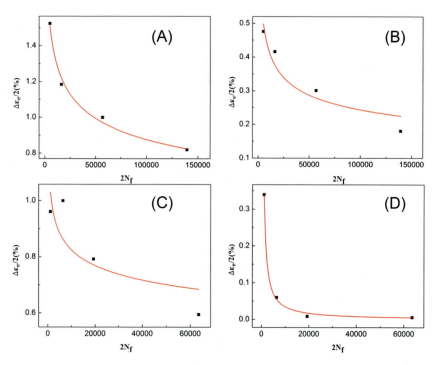

FIGURE 4.22 Low-cycle fatigue deforming relationship curves of TLM alloy. (A) Fitting curve of $\Delta\varepsilon_e/2 \sim 2N$ of TLM with solution treatment. (B) Fitting curve of $\Delta\varepsilon_p/2 \sim 2N$ of TLM with solution treatment. (C) Fitting curve of $\Delta\varepsilon_e/2 \sim 2N$ of TLM with aging treatment. (D) Fitting curve of $\Delta\varepsilon_p/2 \sim 2N$ of TLM with aging treatment.

TABLE 4.28 Fracture toughness of TLM alloy.

No.	K_q (MPa m$^{1/2}$)	Heat treatment
1	101.5	680°C/1 h + 510°C/4 h, AC
2	102.0	
1	118.3	680°C/1 h + 510°C/6 h, AC
2	111.2	
1	117.0	510°C/4 h, AC
2	100.5	
1	132.9	510°C/6 h, AC

AC, Air cooling.

and the number of load reverse cycles is $2N_f$. As is shown in Fig. 4.22, the strain-life relationship of TLM alloy is determined as follows:

$$\text{Solid solution state:} \frac{\Delta \varepsilon t}{2} = 7.126(2Nf)^{-0.812} + 3.857(2Nf)^{-0.240}$$

$$\text{Aging annealed state:} \frac{\Delta \varepsilon t}{2} = 2.076(2Nf)^{-0.1} + 455.32(2Nf)^{-1.03}$$

4.2.8 Dynamic fracture toughness of TLM alloy

Plate specimens with 25 and 30-mm thickness were machined from a rod of Φ90 mm with hot forged and 680°C/1 h + 510°C/4 h, AC heat treatment. The values of the plane strain fracture toughness K_q were 101.5 and 102.0 MPa m$^{1/2}$, as independently tested by two different testing agencies. As shown in Table 4.28, TLM alloy has high fracture toughness values.

4.2.9 Wearability of TLM alloy

Equipment for testing the wear resistance of TLM alloy is shown in Fig. 4.23. The sample is fixed in the center of the instrument, and a spherical pressure head (SiC) rotates around the sample at a speed of 200 revolutions min^{-1}, with a load of 36 g. The samples used were hot rolled TLM alloy with different heat treatment as follows: AC at 750°C/1 h, AC at 680°C/1 h + 510°C/4 h, AC at 680°C/1 h + 510°C/6 h, AC at 510°C/4 h, AC at 510°C/6 h, aging Ti13Nb13Zr, and annealed Ti6Al4V. The samples were 15 × 15 × 1 mm³ plates.

The friction coefficient and the wear resistance of the TLM alloy in different states are shown in Table 4.29 and Fig. 4.24, respectively. For comparison the test results of annealed Ti6Al4V alloys and aging-

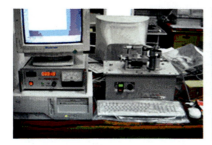
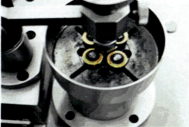

FIGURE 4.23 Wear test instrument.

TABLE 4.29 Friction coefficient of TLM and other biomedical Ti alloys.

Sample	No. 1	No. 2	No. 3	No. 4	No. 5	No. 6	No. 7
Friction coefficient	0.09	0.11	0.14	0.21	0.21	0.21	0.25

Source: *data from Z. Yu, Y. Zheng, J. Niu, Q. Huangfu, Y. Zhang, S. Yu, Microstructure and wear resistance of Ti-3Zr-2Sn-3Mo-15Nb (TLM) alloy, Transactions of Nonferrous Metals Society of China 17 (2007) 495s–499s.*

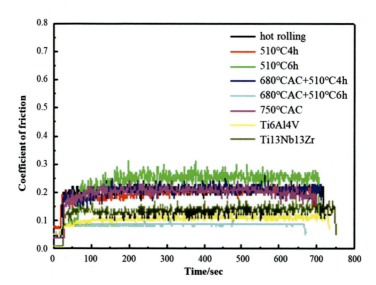

FIGURE 4.24 Friction coefficient curves of TLM and other biomedical Ti alloys. Source: *data from Z. Yu, Y. Zheng, J. Niu, Q. Huangfu, Y. Zhang, S. Yu, Microstructure and wear resistance of Ti-3Zr-2Sn-3Mo-15Nb (TLM) alloy, Transactions of Nonferrous Metals Society of China 17 (2007) 495s–499s.*

treated Ti13Nb13Zr alloys are also presented. It can be seen that the heat treatment system and alloy composition have a great influence on the wear resistance of Ti alloys. The friction coefficient of Ti alloys in different states increases in the following order: TLM with 680°C/1 h, AC + 510°C/6 h AC (No. 1) < Ti6Al4V annealed (No. 2) < Ti13Nb13Zr aging state (No. 3) < TLM hot rolled (No. 4) ≈ TLM with 750°C/1 h, AC + 510°C/4 h (No. 5) ≈ TLM with 510°C/4 h, AC (No. 6) < TLM with 510°C/6 h, AC (No. 7).

Figs. 4.25–4.27 show the surface morphology after the friction test of TLM alloy and its contrast Ti alloy samples. As can be seen from the figures, the scratches in aged Ti13Nb13Zr and annealed Ti6Al4V are relatively shallow and less abrasive after 100 times of amplification. However, after the AC treatment of TLM alloy at 680°C/1 h, AC + 510°C/6 h, the scratches can hardly be seen with the same optical

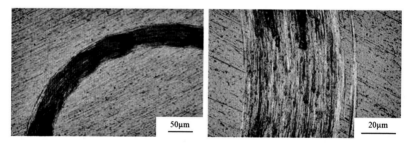

FIGURE 4.25 Wear surface morphology of aging treated Ti13Nb13Zr. *Source: data from Z. Yu, Y. Zheng, J. Niu, Q. Huangfu, Y. Zhang, S. Yu, Microstructure and wear resistance of Ti-3Zr-2Sn-3Mo-15Nb (TLM) alloy, Transactions of Nonferrous Metals Society of China 17 (2007) 495–499.*

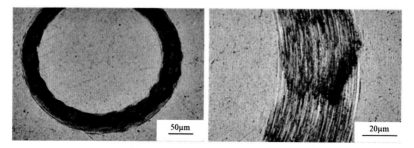

FIGURE 4.26 Wear surface morphology of annealed Ti6Al4V. *Source: data from Z. Yu, Y. Zheng, J. Niu, Q. Huangfu, Y. Zhang, S. Yu, Microstructure and wear resistance of Ti-3Zr-2Sn-3Mo-15Nb (TLM) alloy, Transactions of Nonferrous Metals Society of China 17 (2007) 495–499.*

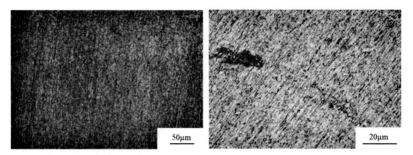

FIGURE 4.27 Wear surface morphology of TLM treated in 680°C/1 h, AC + 510°C/6 h, AC. AC, Air cooling. Source: *data from Z. Yu, Y. Zheng, J. Niu, Q. Huangfu, Y. Zhang, S. Yu, Microstructure and wear resistance of Ti-3Zr-2Sn-3Mo-15Nb (TLM) alloy, Transactions of Nonferrous Metals Society of China 17 (2007) 495–499.*

amplification, and there are very few abrasive particles, which is consistent with the test results of friction coefficient reported earlier [20].

References

[1] L. Luo, Z. Yu, L. Zhou, Mechanical and corrosion properties of near β biomedical titanium alloy, Chinese Journal of Rare Metals 29 (2017) 254–256.
[2] X. Li, X. He, Z. Yu, L. Wang, Ames tests on two new titanium alloys, Rare Metal Materials and Engineering 36 (2007) 489–492.
[3] Z. Xu, Y. Zhang, Z. Wang, Z. Yu, L. Zhou, Y. Zhao, Oral mucous membrane irritation tests on new medical β-type titanium alloys, Rare Metal Materials and Engineering 35 (2006) 110–113.
[4] M. Zhang, Z. Yu, L. Zhou, D. Zhang, Evaluation on biocompatibility of beta-type titanium alloys, Rare Metal Materials and Engineering 36 (2007) 1815–1819.
[5] M. Zhang, Z. Yu, L. Zhou, D. Zhang, Biocompatibility evaluation of β-type titanium alloys, Journal of Clinical Rehabilitative Tissue Engineering Research 14 (2010) 7849–7853.
[6] W. Bing, M. Zhang, Z. Yu, Y. Wen, Z. Ji, Animal experiments of HA coating treated by MAO on porous titanium implants, Chinese Journal of Bone and Joint Injury 26 (2011) 319–321.
[7] W. Jing, J. Han, M. Zhang, H. Cai, Z. Yu, T. Gao, Implantation study of porous β titanium alloy and its MAO coatings, Rare Metal Materials and Engineering 41 (2012) 1657–1660.
[8] Z. Yu, S. Yu, J. Cheng, X. Ma, Development and application of novel biomedical titanium alloy materials, Acta Metallurgica Sinica 53 (2017) 1238–1264.
[9] X. Ma, Y. Han, Z. Yu, Q. Sun, J. Niu, S. Yuan, Phase transformation and mechanical properties of TLM titanium alloy for orthopaedic implant application, Rare Metal Materials and Engineering 41 (2012) 1535–1538.
[10] X. Ma, Z. Yu, Y. Han, X. Song, Q. Sun, In situ scanning electron microscopy observation of deformation and fracture behavior of Ti-3Zr-2Sn-3Mo-25Nb alloy, Rare Metals 31 (2012) 318–322.
[11] Z. Yu, X. Ma, S. Yu, M. Zhang, J. Han, C. Liu, Micro-nano technology and latest progress of biomedical titanium alloy, The Chinese Journal of Nonferrous Metals 20 (2010) 1008–1012.

[12] D. Kent, W. Xiao, G. Wang, Z. Yu, M. Dargusch, Thermal stability of an ultrafine grain β-Ti alloy, Materials Science and Engineering: A 556 (2012) 582–587.
[13] Z. Yu, L. Zhou, L. Luo, M. Fan, Y. Fu, Investigation on mechanical compatibility matching for biomedical titanium alloys, Key Engineering Materials 288 (2005) 595–598.
[14] Z. Yu, L. Zhou, Influence of martensitic transformation on mechanical compatibility of biomedical β type titanium alloy TLM, Materials Science and Engineering: A 438 (2006) 391–394.
[15] Y. Tian, Z. Yu, J. Niu, S. Yu, J. Han, C. Liu, et al., Elastic deformation behavior of Ti-3Zr-2Sn-3Mo-25Nb alloy for biomedical applications, Rare Metal Materials and Engineering 43 (2014) 132–136.
[16] X. Ma, Z. Yu, J. Niu, S. Yu, J. Cheng, Effect of heat treatment on superelasticity in Ti-3Zr-2Sn-3Mo-25Nb Alloy, Rare Metal Materials and Engineering 45 (2016) 1588–1592.
[17] Z. Yu, Y. Zheng, J. Niu, B. Wang, Q. Huangfu, Y. Zhang, et al., Shape memory effect and superelastic properties of novel Ti-3Zr-2Sn-3Mo-15Nb alloy, Journal of Functional Materials 38 (2007) 3126–3129.
[18] Z. Yu, Y. Zheng, L. Zhou, B. Wang, J. Niu, H. Qiang, et al., Shape memory effect and superelastic property of a novel Ti-3Zr-2Sn-3Mo-15Nb alloy, Rare Metal Materials and Engineering 37 (2008) 1–5.
[19] Z. Yu, G. Wang, X. Ma, Y. Zhang, M. Dargusch, Shape memory characteristics of a near β titanium alloy, Materials Science and Engineering: A 513 (2009) 233–238.
[20] Z. Yu, Y. Zheng, J. Niu, Q. Huangfu, Y. Zhang, S. Yu, Microstructure and wear resistance of Ti-3Zr-2Sn-3Mo-15Nb (TLM) alloy, Transactions of Nonferrous Metals Society of China 17 (2007) s495–s499.

CHAPTER 5

Surface modification and functionalization of TLM alloy

5.1 Surface modification of Ti alloys

The issues of surface or interface of metal surgical implants are crucial. The surface characteristics are directly related to the biochemical reaction between the metal substrate and body tissues, and their interaction also determine the success of artificial prosthetic devices in *in-vivo* therapy and rehabilitation. The interface is a core and hotspot issue for metal materials with biocoating. The surface and interface characteristics determine the final comprehensive performance of materials. Because of differences in the therapeutic purposes of surgical implants and the surrounding biological environments in which they are placed, the purposes of surface modification and the corresponding methods are diverse. For example, for artificial prostheses of hard tissues such as bone and teeth, we should consider how to achieve osseointegration as early as possible and maintain the long-term effect of this combination. For cardiovascular stents we should consider how to inhibit in-stent thrombosis and restenosis.

At present, the surface modification methods of biomedical Ti and its alloys can be categorized as chemical methods, physical methods, and mechanical methods according to the surface characteristics of the metal and the formation mechanisms of the modified coatings (films).

Chemical methods involve the use of chemical reactions to treat the surface of Ti and its alloys, including conventional chemical treatment, electrochemical treatment, the sol—gel process, chemical vapor deposition (CVD), and biochemical decoration. The chemical treatment mainly depends on the chemical reactions that occur at the interface between the Ti substrate and the solution, commonly including alkaline heat treatment, hydrogen peroxide solution treatment, and passivation treatment. The sol−gel technology is widely used in the preparation of bioceramic films such as Ti dioxide coatings, calcium phosphate coatings, Ti dioxide/hydroxyapatite (HA) composite coatings, silicon coatings, etc. Electrochemical treatment includes anodic oxidation (AO) and microarc oxidation (MAO). The CVD technology mainly realizes the deposition of a layer of nonvolatile stable compounds on the Ti surface *via* a chemical reaction between the vapor phase and the Ti substrate, such as the preparation of hard diamond-like carbon films by CVD technology. Biochemical decoration aims to fix peptides, proteins, or growth factors onto the surface of the Ti substrate, hence inducing special reactions of cells and tissues. Nowadays, there are many technologies to decorate the surface of Ti and its alloys, such as silanization, self-assembled monolayers, and protein anchoring.

In the physical methods, no chemical reaction occurs during the surface modification process. When the physical methods are used for surface treatment, the formation of the surface layers of Ti and its alloys are mainly attributed to heat, kinetic energy, electric energy, and so on. Physical methods mainly include various spraying technologies (e.g., thermal, plasma, arc and flame spraying), physical vapor deposition (e.g., magnetron sputtering, arc ion plating), glow discharge plasma implantation, and laser etching. These methods are used to consolidate different metal or ceramic particles on the surface to form bioactive coatings (films) with a micro-scale or nano-scale structure whose chemical composition is the same as or different from that of the substrate. The main characteristics of the bioactive coatings (films) are that the size of the micro-scale or nano-scale grains is relatively uniform, there is an obvious interface between the surface layer and the substrate, and the thickness and grain size of the modified layer can be regulated by changing the process parameters, but the dimensions of materials slightly increase compared to those before the treatment. The key to this technology is achieving a strong bonding between the surface layer and the substrate and between the microparticles or nanoparticles of surface layer, thereby ensuring that no grain growth occurs in the surface layer.

The mechanical methods involve the treatment or preforming of the material surface by mechanical processing methods, such as surface cutting, grinding, polishing, and sandblasting, and their main purpose is to obtain special surface morphology with microstructure or nanostructure, different roughness, or some other requirement. Compared to conventional coarse-grained materials, nanomaterials have excellent physical and chemical properties. The special surface structure of Ti alloys that form after micronization or nanoization is conducive to the adhesion, differentiation, and proliferation of cells *in vivo*. Two common mechanical methods have been developed: surface self-micronization or nanoization and the hybrid method. In surface self-micronization or nanoization for polycrystalline materials, the nonequilibrium treatment method can increase the surface roughness and free energy of the material, and gradually refine the original coarse-grained structure to the micro-scale or nano-scale level. The main characteristics are that the grain size gradually increases along the thickness direction. There is no obvious interface between the nanolayer and the substrate. The dimensions of materials do not change much compared to those before the treatment. At present, surface mechanical processing and nonequilibrium thermodynamics are the two main methods to achieve the surface micronization or nanoization *via* the nonequilibrium processes. In the hybrid method, microcrystalline or nanocrystalline solid solutions or compounds consisting of different components from the matrix are formed on the surface layer of the nanostructured materials by combining the surface nanocrystallization technology with a chemical treatment. This method is more practical because the advantages of the two methods are combined.

In the past ten years the improvement of biological properties of metal materials by micronization or nanoization of surface grains has been numerously studies and reported. The preparation of a layer of nanocrystals on the Ti surface by the surface plastic deformation method for the bioactivity modification has attracted great interest from biomaterials researchers. It points out a new direction for the optimization and upgrades of the mechanical properties of conventional biomedical metal materials and is also the best way to solve the current problems of low strength, high modulus, and poor biomechanical properties of biomedical commercial pure Ti (CP−Ti). For example, the nanocrystalline CP−Ti was fabricated by a high-pressure torsion method, and the *in vitro* biological results showed that it can significantly promote the adhesion and viability of preosteoblast cells on its surface [1]. The nanocrystalline CP−Ti was prepared by the hydrostatic extrusion technology, and the research results also showed that grain refinement affects the adsorption behavior of proteins and that the nanostructure benefits the adhesion and proliferation of SaOS-2 cells [2]. Zhang's research group successfully fabricated an ultrafine-grained nanocrystalline surface layer on the surface of CP−Ti and Ti6Al4V (TC4) alloy, using the sliding friction treatment (SFT). *In vitro* tests proved that the hydrophilicity of the prepared fine-grained surface layer was greatly improved, more human osteoblasts adhered to the surface of the finer-grained materials, and the treatment of TC4 alloy by SFT could promote the collagen secretion and extracellular matrix mineralization of osteoblasts [3,4] as shown in Fig. 5.1.

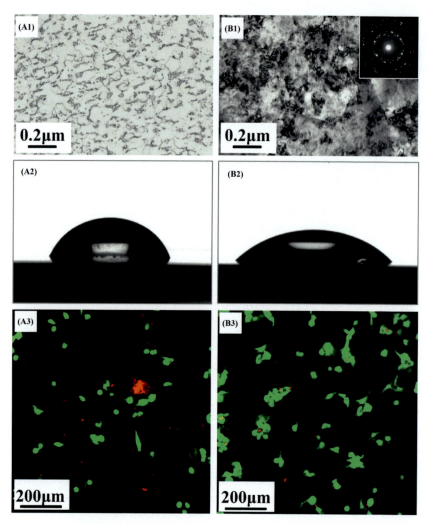

FIGURE 5.1 Morphology of TC4 ally with (A1) coarse grains and (B1) fine grains and the corresponding (A2, B2) hydrophilicity and (A3, B3) cell adhesion on its surface.

5.2 Surface functionalization of Ti alloys

5.2.1 Surface bioactive modification of metals for repairing bones/teeth hard tissues

The bioactive composite coatings on the metal surface are effective ways to solve the poor osseointegration of the metal substrate and bone tissue in the early stage. The micromechanism is that the bioactive coatings induce the growth of bonelike apatite on its surface, and then this bone apatite bonds with the new bone *via* chemical bonding, thereby achieving firm bonding between the metal and bone tissue. In terms of chemical composition, three main types of bioactive coating have been developed: (1) chemical soluble ceramics, such as bioglass, calcium silicate, and HA; (2) chemical insoluble ceramics, such as Ti oxide, zirconium oxide, and calcium carbonate; and (3) organic polymers that are rich in −COOH and −PO$_4$H$_2$, which are not suitable for coatings on metals because of their low strength and poor structural stability. The higher the biological activity of the coating material, the shorter is the time for osseointegration (i.e., forming synostosis with bone) in the body.

HA coating is the only bioactive coating that has been approved by the U.S. Food and Drug Administration (FDA) and used commercially. To ensure the long-term structural integrity of the coating and metal after implantation in the human body, the quality requirements of the FDA and ISO international standards for HA coatings used in orthopedics and dentistry are as follows: crystallinity greater than 62%, phase purity greater than 95%, bonding strength greater than 50 MPa, and thickness of 50−75 μm [5]. However, clinical applications show that the longest life of HA coatings whose properties meet the FDA and ISO standards is only 8 years, and the osseointegration still takes a long time (3 months) [6]. Therefore the development of new bioactive coatings should not only further improve its early osseointegration ability, but also strive to improve the bonding strength and the long-term stability of the structure within the life span.

To improve the biological activity of HA coatings, SrHA (Sr partially substitutes for Ca in HA) coatings, SiHA (SiO$_4^{3−}$ partially substitutes for PO$_4^{3−}$ in HA) coatings, and decoration of coatings by biological molecular RGD peptide have recently been developed. Studies showed that both the SrHA [7] and SiHA coatings [8] have higher abilities to induce bonelike apatite, cell adhesion, and function expression effects in comparison HA coating, and the RGD peptides that are grafted onto the surface of Ti-based materials with long-chain polymers (e.g., polyethylene glycol) show higher osteoblast attachment and calcification rates [9]. However, the long-term effectiveness of these new soluble coatings *in vivo*, the bonding after complete degradation, and the bonding mechanism are the scientific issues that need to be explored. These are the theoretical bases for the structure design and function construction of the coatings.

Considering the long-term stability of coatings, TiO$_2$ and CaTiO$_3$ with better chemical stability than HA have received much attention in recent years. Studies have found that amorphous TiO$_2$ and coarse-grained do not have the ability to induce the bone apatite, while nanocrystalline TiO$_2$ does. However, there is still a lack of consensus on the osseointegration ability of these coatings compared to the HA coating. Recent studies have shown that the chemically slightly soluble $CaTiO_3$ coating has good abilities to induce the bony apatite and for osteoblast adhesion and functional expression [10]. However, its stability in the physiological environment and effects on the formation and osseointegration of new bone have not been determined.

The formation of new bone on the surface of surgical implants is controlled by the response effect of various cells (e.g., osteoblasts, osteoclasts, fibroblasts, macrophages) on the prosthesis surface. The response effect of various cells to the implants is related not only to the surface chemical composition of materials, but also to the micro-scale or nano-scale of the surface configuration. After studying the response selectivity of different cells to the microconfiguration and nanoconfiguration on the material surface, Mendonça et al. [11] pointed out that nanocrystalline materials can inhibit the adhesion of fibroblasts while promoting the adhesion of osteoblasts. Richert et al. [12] believed that the nanoporous configuration can inhibit the growth of fibroblasts while promoting the growth of osteoblasts, but it is not selective for the attachment of these two kinds of cells. It can be concluded that the present studies lack consensus on the rules and micromechanisms of the attachment of different cells selected by the nanoconfiguration of the material surface, and the law of the simultaneous interaction between multiple cells in the organism and implants needs to be further explored [13].

In view of the contradiction between the early osseointegration ability of the single-phase bioactive coatings and their long-term stability, from the summarization of the research progress of the biofunctionalization modification of hard bone tissue implants, it can be seen that multiple sets of nanostructured coatings with selectivity of biological response is the development trend of bioactive coatings. The challenges are how to further improve the early osseointegration ability and long-term stability of the bioactive modified layer and how to selectively control the interface reaction.

5.2.2 Anticoagulant surface modification for cardiovascular stents

In-stent thrombosis and restenosis are common problems in the clinical applications of metal vascular stents. The bare metal cardiovascular stents have poor anticoagulation, high sensitization and inflammation, and a high in-stent restenosis rate of 20%−35% [14]. As a result, various coatings have been developed: (1) Inorganic inert coatings, such as DLC, Ta_2O_5, Nb_2O_5, SiC, Ti(N,C), TaN, and TiNO, can inhibit the dissolution of metal ions, improve anticoagulation, and reduce thrombosis.

However, TiNO can reduce the restenosis rate to 15%, whereas the others have no obvious effect on inhibiting restenosis caused by excessive intimal proliferation [14]. (2) Polymer coatings loaded with antiproliferative drug inhibits the proliferation of vascular smooth muscle cells by the local release of drugs (e.g., rapamycin, paclitaxel), thereby inhibiting restenosis caused by intimal hyperplasia and showing better early and midterm safety. However, these drugs also inhibit the endothelialization of the stent wall while inhibiting vascular intimal hyperplasia. The polymers on the stent surface will still cause late thrombosis after the complete release of drugs, and there is still a certain possibility of late restenosis [15]. (3) Surface modification methods such as ion implantation can effectively improve the blood compatibility of stents by surface decoration [16].

Endothelialization of the stent surface is the most effective way to inhibit thrombosis and restenosis [17]. There are two main ways to promote rapid endothelialization of the stent surface. The first method is inoculation of endothelial repair cells *in vitro* such as endothelial cells and mesenchymal stem cells. But this presents problems, such as fewer sources of seed cells and difficult storage of endothelialized stents. The second method of promoting rapid endothelialization is induction of endothelialization *in vivo*. Studies have shown that the bioactive components such as RGD peptides, endothelial cell growth factor, etc. coated in stent can promote the repair of damaged vascular endothelial cells [18], and the nanoconfiguration on the stent surface can promote the growth and proliferation of endothelial cells. Consequently, the loading of drugs or bioactive components with inorganic nanoporous coatings will be the important development direction of drug-eluting stents in the future.

Ti alloys are the main raw materials for heart valves, vascular stents, and other devices that come into contact with human blood. Extensive experiments proved that implantation of the bare stents in the blood vessel induced the activation of endothelial cell growth factor, which leads to the proliferation and migration of endothelial cells, then induces the proliferation of smooth muscle cells, and eventually results in thrombosis and the restenosis of the stent. However, the micromechanisms of in-stent restenosis still need further studies, and the probable influencing factors include the thrombosis formation, intimal hyperplasia, inflammatory response, and vascular remodeling. Since there are obvious hemodynamic changes in the process of the extension and expansion during the implantation of metal stents and the subsequent intimal hyperplasia and vascular remodeling process, the mechanical microenvironment changes during the vascular stent implantation and the materials surface characteristics should be combined to study the surface-interface reactions and the law of interaction between metal, biomodified coating, and cells so as to clarify the micromechanisms of secondary restenosis in the late stage of vascular stent implantation. These are the key scientific problems that need to be addressed immediately for the biofunctionalization surface modification of the cardiovascular stents. The challenges are how to multifunctionalize the surface of the metal stents to endow the stent surface with functions such as anticoagulation, antiinflammatory, and antiintimal hyperplasia properties; the ability to induce endothelialization; and the structural bionic design and construction principles of the stent surface coatings that can actively induce endothelialization [19].

5.2.3 Wear-resistant surface modification of metals for replacement of hard tissues

The aseptic loosening of the joint stem caused by the wear particles generated by the wear of the metal joint head and socket (acetabulum) is a bottleneck problem that has not yet been completely resolved in clinical applications. For example, 6 and 10 years after metal total hip replacement, the aseptic loosening rate is still as high as 5% and 10%, respectively [20], and the existing consensus is that the wear rate is related to the osteolysis caused by the interaction of wear debris particles and macrophages. Hence the improvement of the wear resistance of metal joint head and socket components *via* surface modification to reduce the amount of wear debris is likely to be an effective way to inhibit osteolysis and overcome the aseptic loosening [19,21,22]. In addition, the micromechanisms of aseptic loosening caused by the wear debris and particles also need further study and exploration.

Biomechanical studies showed that thick coatings with low elastic modulus can significantly improve the stress transfer between metals with high elastic modulus, such as biomedical stainless steels and cobalt-chromium alloys, and bone tissue. For example, the mechanical compatibility between artificial joint prostheses and bone is expected to be improved by compositing porous metal coatings with appropriate thicknesses on the dense metal surface. However, the existing bioactive coatings are only osteoconductive but not osteoinductive. Recent studies found that the osteoinductive materials should be a three-dimensional porous structure with open pores with pore sizes more than 100 μm in diameter and whose inner pore walls demonstrate microporous or nanoporous morphology. Porous materials can significantly improve the materials' bond strength with bone by inducing the adhesion and growth of bone tissue in the pores [23]. However, how to give the porous metal coatings high interface adhesive strength and cohesive strength with the metal substrate while having an elastic modulus matching that of bone and how to activate the porous metal coatings to endow good properties such as high osteoinductivity are key problems that needs further research and exploration.

Bacterial infection is another important reason for the failure of surgical implants. The rates of orthopedic and cardiovascular implants' failure caused by bacterial infection reach 4.3%−7.4% [24]. The reason is that bacteria in the body adhere to the implant surface earlier than cells, form biofilms, and result in gangrene in the surrounding bone tissue. Therefore the incorporation of antibacterial or bactericidal components in the bioactive wear-resistance coatings is an effective way to prevent bone tissue gangrene and promote early osseointegration between artificial prostheses and bone. At present, the major methods of antibacterial treatment of biomedical metal surfaces include synthesis of the HA coating containing silver ions, copper ions, fluoride ions, or antibacterial polymer particles; physically embedding in the polymers or covalently grafting of silver ions on the polymers [24]; and grafting of antibacterial polymers and drugs onto the surface of the Ti oxide coating [25]. However, further work is needed to study the dosage of the antibacterial components in the coating and their effects on healthy tissues and cells, how to control the release rate of the antibacterial components to achieve short-term high-efficiency antibacterial and long-term antibacterial effects, and whether the nanoconfiguration of coatings selectively control the attachment of bacteria and normal tissue cells.

Artificial joint materials are required to have sufficient hardness and wear resistance; otherwise, the prostheses will loosen and fail prematurely as a result of frequent fretting and wear. For the low surface hardness and relatively poor wear resistance of biomedical Ti alloys, the current preparation methods of wear-resistant coatings mainly include thermal spraying, electroplating and chemical plating, physical vapor deposition, ion implantation, magnetron sputtering, MAO, and combined surface treatment technologies. The commonly used wear-resistant surface coatings include diamond-like carbon film and Ti nitride (TiN) coating. Among them, the ion implantation technology not only can improve the surface hardness and reduce the surface friction coefficient of Ti alloys, but also can further functionalize the surface. In β-Ti alloys such as TLM, the elements, including Zr, Nb, and Ta, can easily form the hard surface oxide films such as ZrO_2, Nb_2O_3, and Ta_2O_5, respectively. The dense surface can inhibit the dissolution of metal ions and improve the corrosion resistance. The improved surface hardness also enhances the protection ability and wear resistance of the original TiO_2 film. Previous studies showed that the elastic modulus of Ti alloys after ultrafine grain or nanocrystallization treatment is reduced and closer to the elastic modulus of cortical bone. Their hardness is also enhanced to a certain extent, which reduces the generation of wear debris on the bone joint surface, thereby improving the biomechanical compatibility of Ti alloys. Hence the application of surface microtechnology and nanotechnology to the friction and wear contact interface of artificial joints, dental implants, and bone joints will be conducive to delay the occurrence of prosthesis loosening [19].

5.3 Surface dealloying of TLM alloy

Both research and clinical tests found that surface modification technologies such as MAO and electrochemical deposition can obviously improve the biological properties of porous Ti and accelerate osseointegration. However, these research methods all involve additive coatings, which have the risk of coating delamination, adding an interface between the implants and tissue, making the healing process relatively slow and complicated. Consequently, the noncoating surface modification technology has become an important research and development direction. Dealloying is a subtractive or noncoating surface modification technology that reduces the risk of coating delamination and can also improve the biocompatibility of the substrate materials and direct connection between the new bone tissue and implant substrate. Electrochemical dealloying is an advanced surface modification technology to prepare spongelike homogeneous nanoporous metals and their alloys. The multidimensional open micropores formed by this technology are beneficial to the barrier-free transportation of fluid medium molecules. In this continuous microstructure the three-dimensional pores and the framework are completely interlaced with each other. The framework structure can provide mechanical stability for the porous material, whereas the pores provide electronic channels for the catalytically active sites. So far, the reported nanoporous metal foams are all prepared by binary and ternary alloy systems, and the alloys are single-phase solid solutions in the entire composition range. Nanoporous precious metals such as Au and Ag and their alloys were successfully prepared from precursor alloys such as Cu−Pt and Au−Ag−Pt, respectively, while nanoporous foamed Ti and its alloys have many biological functions due to the existence of continuous open pores and will have great potential applications in biomedical devices and other fields. The schematic diagram of the dealloying process of binary alloys is shown in Fig. 5.2.

At present, the dealloying methods that are used domestically and abroad are mainly divided into three types: chemical dealloying, electrochemical dealloying, and molten metal dealloying. The chemical dealloying method is to immerse the alloy in a corrosive solution. The solution type, ion concentration, and temperature are the important

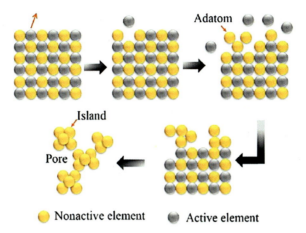

FIGURE 5.2 Schematic diagram of the dealloying process of binary alloys. Source: *data from F. Yang, Electrochemical dealloying synthesis of surface-porous magnesium-aluminum alloys, Taiyuan University of Technology, 2018.*

influencing factors, affecting the diffusion of active elements in the alloy and the surface structure that is finally formed. The electrochemical dealloying method is to use the alloy as an electrode and apply a constant potential as the driving force to achieve the selective dissolution of the active components, in which the applied voltage is the decisive factor. The molten metal dealloying method refers to the use of liquid metal as the dissolution medium and affects the result of dealloying *via* temperature and liquid metal properties, but this method is limited to the preparation of single-hole structures. Theoretically, it is possible to remove the alloying elements of two different phases in binary alloys, leading to the formation of a layered porous structure, but this is not always the case because kinetic factors can change the microstructure evolution process [26]. For example, increasing the temperature or time of chemical dealloying can enhance the diffusion of noble metal elements, but the accelerated coarsening may transform the bimodal porous structure into a uniform porous structure. For electrochemical dealloying, in most cases, the dealloying process and the obtained microstructure can be predicted by the applied potential or driving force.

Sen Yu and Zhentao Yu at the Northwest Institute for Nonferrous Metal Research (NIN) successfully prepared nano-scale microholes on the surface of Ti6Al4V, TLM, and TiNi biomedical Ti alloys *via* dealloying. This research group also successfully fabricated uniform nano-scale pores with different pore diameters and micro-nano hierarchical porous structures by dealloying the surface of the novel TLM alloy. Fig. 5.3 shows the scanning electron microscope (SEM) morphology of the TLM alloy surface after dealloying at different voltages. It can be seen that a uniformly distributed nanoporous surface structure can be obtained after dealloying, and the smallest pore size is around 20 nm and can be controlled by the parameters such as dealloying voltage and time.

The biocompatibility of dealloyed TLM alloy was evaluated by the coculture of osteoblasts (MC3T3-E1), and the statistical results are shown in Fig. 5.4. Compared to the blank control group, the nanoporous structure on the material surface after incubation for 1, 3, and 5 days is obviously more conducive to cell proliferation, and the cell proliferation rates are greater than those of the blank control group, indicating that the nanoporous surface after dealloying has a better ability to promote cell proliferation.

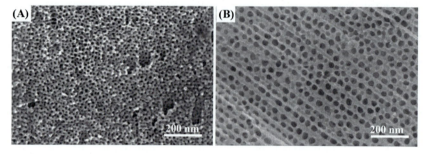

FIGURE 5.3 SEM micrographs of TLM after the dealloying treatment at different voltages. (A) 1 V. (B) 10 V.

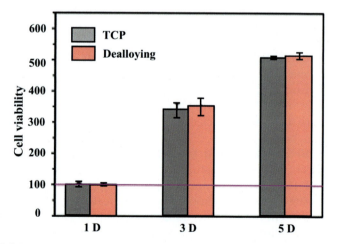

FIGURE 5.4 Cell proliferation rates of each group at different times.

5.4 Bioactive coatings on TLM alloy

Ti and its alloys have become the most promising metallic biomaterials because of their excellent biocompatibility, corrosion resistance, and outstanding comprehensive mechanical properties [19]. However, clinical studies have found that Ti and its alloys are biologically inert in the body, unable to bond with host tissues, and are prone to loosen, leading to surgical failure. Additionally, metal ions produced as a result of physiological corrosion can also cause toxic side effects. One of the major methods to solve these problems is to prepare bioactive coatings on the Ti substrate surface. The application of MAO technology to the surface modification of Ti alloys has emerged as a hotspot research direction in the past 20 years. This technology has many advantages, including simple process, high efficiency, no restriction of the workpiece surface shape, and high bond strength between the coating and substrate [27,28]. In addition, adjustment of the electrolyte can make the film formed rich in calcium and phosphorous elements similar to the composition of human bone tissue, which can promote the growth of osteoblasts on the film surface, and the dense MAO film can further improve the anticorrosion properties and wear resistance of the Ti substrate [29,30]. This section mainly introduces the preparation of the porous bioactive films on the surface of the novel near β Ti alloy TLM and studies and evaluates the phase composition, surface microstructure, and bioactivity of the oxide films.

5.4.1 Preparation of porous bioactive coatings by microarc oxidation

Three different MAO test process are selected for the deposition of coatings: common MAO, multiphase MAO, and ultraviolet irradiation MAO. Common MAO is used to perform MAO treatment of the TLM alloy in a water-based electrolyte with pulsed direct current power supply at a voltage of 250 to 500 V with a duty cycle of 50%. The treatment time is 10−15 minutes, and the temperature of the electrolyte is kept below 40°C with the TLM alloy sample as the anode and stainless steel as the cathode. In multiphase MAO, Ti alloys are treated in electrolyte prepared from calcium acetate and sodium glycerophosphate. Other parameters are the same as those used in the common MAO process. Ultraviolet irradiation MAO involves the same process as that of common MAO, but after the films have been prepared, they are exposed to ultraviolet light for radiation treatment. The center wavelength of ultraviolet light is 253.7 nm, and the power density is 65 $\mu W\ cm^{-2}$.

The X-ray diffraction (XRD) curves of the three types of MAO films on the TLM alloy are shown in Fig. 5.5. It can be seen that except for a

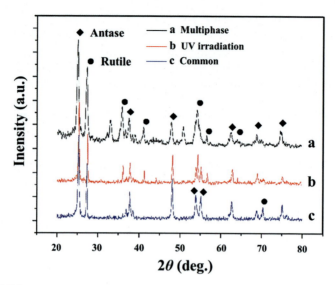

FIGURE 5.5 XRD patterns of the three different films prepared by MAO. *XRD*, X-ray diffraction; *MAO*, microarc oxidation.

few impurity peaks, the coating is mainly composed of rutile TiO$_2$, anatase TiO$_2$, and a small amount of amorphous phase, among which rutile TiO$_2$ accounts for the largest proportion. This is because the MAO films are produced at a very high voltage, and the instantaneous temperature can reach more than 2000°C, which is higher than the phase transition temperature of rutile. The diffraction peaks are sharp and narrow without broadening or splitting, indicating that the films have high crystallinity and that the atoms in the crystalline TiO$_2$ films have preferred orientation and are regularly arranged.

However, no obvious calcium-phosphorus compound phase is observed from the XRD spectra. According to the analysis, there may be two reasons: (1) The instantaneous temperature in the microarc area during the MAO process is very high, and the existence time of each arc point is 10–15 μs, whereas the temperature of the MAO treatment liquid is only tens of degrees, the cooling rate of the molten materials is extremely high when they are solidified, and their degree of supercooling is also extremely large. Therefore the calcium-phosphorus compounds tend to exist in an amorphous form in the films. (2) Each arc point of MAO means a micromolten pool, in which calcium and phosphorus elements participate in complex high-temperature metallurgical reactions but do not form a large amount of calcium-phosphorus compounds. They are dissolved in Ti oxide in the form of solid solution or exist in the form of various metallic or nonmetallic inclusions, which are not obviously displayed, owing to the small amount of each.

Fig. 5.6 displays the SEM images of the typical MAO films on the TLM alloy surface. The surface of the three kinds of MAO TiO$_2$ films are covered with micropores as a result of the passageway for the formation of electric sparks during microarc discharge. The films have uniform thicknesses, and the porous film layer is continuous, dense, and integrated without peeling and wide cracks. Compared to the film prepared by the multiphase process, the common MAO film has a smoother surface and more regular micropore shapes, but there are a few granular solids on the surface of the multiphase MAO film, which may result from the generation of other calcium-phosphorus compounds besides TiO$_2$ during the MAO process. There is no obvious difference between the surface of the ultraviolet irradiated film and that of the common MAO film.

The contact angles of the three coatings were tested by the hydrophilicity test, and the statistical results are shown in Table 5.1. It can be seen that the contact angle of the TiO$_2$ active film prepared by the ultraviolet irradiation process with distilled water is the smallest. The photoinduced superhydrophilicity of the TiO$_2$ surface originates from the change of its surface structure [31]. TiO$_2$ is an n-type semiconductor, its band gap of anatase is 3.2 eV, and the wavelength is about 380 nm. Under ultraviolet light with a wavelength shorter than 380 nm, the

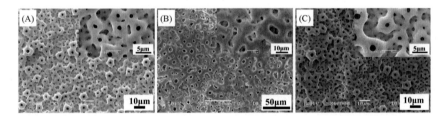

FIGURE 5.6 SEM micrographs of the MAO films. (A) Common technology. (B) Multiphase technology. (C) Ultraviolet irradiation technology. *SEM*, Scanning electron microscope; *MAO*, microarc oxidation.

TABLE 5.1 Contact angles of three kinds of microarc oxidation (MAO) films.

Surface treatment	Contact angle (degree)			Average value (degree)
	1	2	3	
Common MAO	45.3	46.1	44.8	45.4
Multiphase MAO	44.2	44.9	43.2	44.1
Ultraviolet irradiation MAO	11.1	10.8	10.9	11.6

valence band electrons of TiO_2 are excited to the conduction band. Electrons and holes migrate to the surface, electrons react with Ti^{4+}, and holes react with oxygen ions on the surface to form Ti^{3+} and oxygen vacancies, respectively. At this time, water in the air dissociates and adsorbs in the oxygen vacancies and becomes chemisorbed water (hydroxyl, OH^-, belongs to a hydrophilic group, which is easy to physically adsorb water to form hydrogen bonds and thus enhances the hydrophilicity of the materials surface), which is also the reason why the contact angle of the sample greatly reduces after the UV activation in this test. Chemisorbed water can further adsorb moisture in the air to form a physical adsorption layer. As a result, highly hydrophilic microdomains are formed around the Ti^{3+} defects, while the surface residual area remains hydrophobic. The hydrophilic and hydrophobic regions with nano size and uniform distribution are formed on the surface of TiO_2, which is similar to the phenomenon of the two-dimensional capillary phenomenon. Because the size of the water droplets is much larger than the area of the hydrophilic regions, the macroscopic performance is that the contact angle of water on its surface becomes smaller.

Since the hydrophilicity and free energy of the material surface are closely related to the absorption and denaturation of blood components, the increase in hydrophilicity of the material surface, and thus reduction in the surface free energy to the surface free energy value, which is close to that of the vascular intima, will be beneficial to improve the antithrombotic performance of the material and the blood compatibility of the surface of intervention or implant material.

5.4.2 Preparation of strontium-containing bioactive coatings by microarc oxidation

Strontium-containing bioactive coating is prepared on the TLM alloy in a water-based electrolyte prepared from strontium acetate, calcium acetate, and sodium glycerophosphate by using a pulsed power supply under the conditions of a voltage of 300 V, a duty cycle of 26%, and a frequency of 100 Hz, followed by 1 hour of ultraviolet irradiation in simulated body fluid (SBF) solution or deionized water.

The coating synthesized by MAO process mainly consists of anatase TiO_2 and rutile TiO_2, its bonding strength is approximately 44.2 MPa, and the phase composition and surface morphology of the coating do not change after ultraviolet light irradiation. After soaking in the SBF solution for 9 days, the coating can induce the formation of bone apatite, which covers the original porous surface of the coating and shows good bioactivity, as shown in Figs. 5.7 and 5.8.

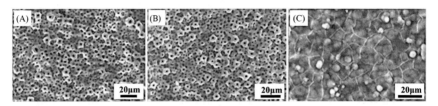

FIGURE 5.7 Surface morphology of the MAO coating (A) before and (B) after ultraviolet irradiation in SBF. (C) The ultraviolet irradiated MAO coating after 9-day immersion in SBF. *MAO*, Microarc oxidation; *SBF*, simulated body fluid.

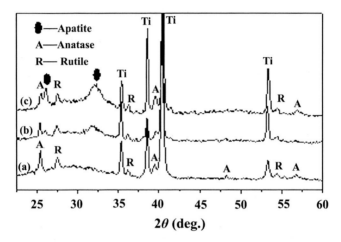

FIGURE 5.8 XRD spectra of the ultraviolet irradiated MAO sample (A) before and after being soaked in SBF for (B) 6 and (C) 9 days. *XRD*, X-ray diffraction; *MAO*, microarc oxidation; *SBF*, simulated body fluid.

5.4.3 Preparation of barium titanate bioactive coatings by microarc oxidation

Previous studies proved that weak current can stimulate bone formation and promote bone healing. However, none of the existing bioactive coatings can form electrical stimulation in the body. Therefore the barium titanate coating was prepared on the TLM surface by MAO to make use of the unique piezoelectric effect of barium titanate. The detailed preparation process is that the Ti alloy is subjected to the MAO treatment for 1 hour with a pulsed power supply at a voltage of 80 V, a duty cycle of 26%, and a frequency of 100 Hz in electrolyte composed of 0.06 M $Ba(OH)_2 \cdot 8H_2O$ and 0.4 mol/L NaOH. A pure barium titanate coating with a thickness of about 35 μm was synthesized. The adhesion strength of the coating is about 36 MPa, and the coating after polarization can induce the formation of bone apatite after soaking in the SBF solution for 10 days, as shown in Fig. 5.9.

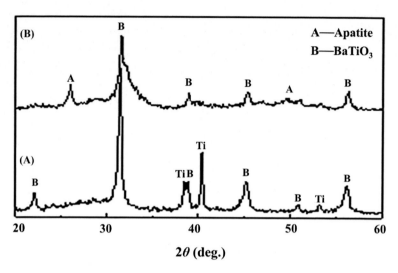

FIGURE 5.9 XRD patterns of the barium titanate coatings prepared by MAO (A) before and (B) after immersion in the SBF solution for 10 days. *XRD*, X-ray diffraction; *MAO*, microarc oxidation; *SBF*, simulated body fluid.

5.4.4 Preparation of TiO$_2$ nanotube bioactive films by anodic oxidation

TLM alloy discs with a thickness of 1 mm and a diameter of 14.5 mm were used as the anode, and a platinum plate was used as the cathode. The coating fabrication was conducted in an electrolyte solution containing 1 vol.% HF + 3 vol.% HNO$_3$ at a voltage of 10–30 V for 2 hours by using a common AO apparatus. After AO, some samples were carried out at 550°C for 2 hours in air for the heat treatment. The irregularly arranged TiO$_2$ nanotube arrays (thin films) appeared on the TLM surface as depicted in Fig. 5.10. As shown in Fig. 5.11A, some globular sediments are seen on the surface of the TiO$_2$ thin film after 3-day immersion in the SBF solution. The EDS spectrum in Fig. 5.11B shows a certain intensity of the HA diffraction peaks and higher contents of the Ca and P elements, which proves that the TiO$_2$ nanotube arrays can induce the formation of HA with an inorganic component similar to that of natural bone. The apatite can be induced by the irregular TiO$_2$ nanotube arrays formed on the TLM alloy surface in SBF, which means that the TiO$_2$ nanotube arrays may absorb the calcium and phosphorous ions in the body, inducing the deposition of bioactive apatite.

Fig. 5.12 presents SEM images of the osteoblasts after incubation on the surface of the TLM alloy for 24 hours. The osteoblasts spread well and display fusiform, irregular polygons on the surface of the Ti plate

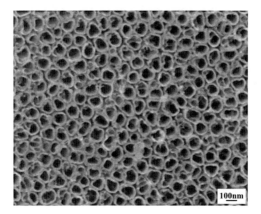

FIGURE 5.10 FE-SEM micrographs of the TiO$_2$ nanotube arrays formed on the TLM alloy. *FE-SEM*, Field emission scanning electron microscope.

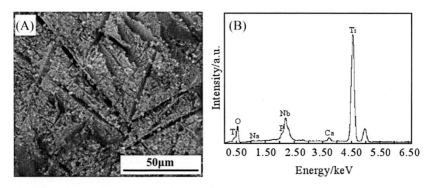

FIGURE 5.11 (A) FE-SEM micrographs and (B) EDS spectrum of the TiO$_2$ nanotubes arrays on the TLM alloy after being soaked in SBF for 3 days. *FE-SEM*, Field emission scanning electron microscope; *EDS*, energy dispersive spectroscopy; *SBF*, simulated body fluid.

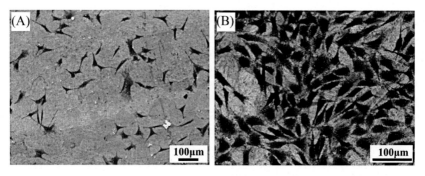

FIGURE 5.12 FE-SEM micrographs of the early cell attachment rate of osteoblasts cultured for 24 hours on the TiO$_2$ nanotube arrays, (A) on the Ti and (B) on TLM substrate. *FE-SEM*, Field emission scanning electron microscope.

with the TiO$_2$ nanotube arrays. Some osteoblasts demonstrate a radiating shape. As a whole, the TiO$_2$ nanotube arrays are uniform and crack-free and macroscopically demonstrate an ordered porous structure, which causes the surface of TLM alloy to increase notably and then improves the attachment strength of cells on its surface. In the meantime, the TiO$_2$ nanotube arrays provide favorable anchor sites for the adhesion of osteoblasts. Once cells adhere prematurely, they will send an appropriate adhesion signal to guide the adhesion of the remaining osteoblasts.

It has also been found that the irregularly oriented TiO$_2$ nanotube arrays on the surface of TLM after the treatment of AO can accelerate the deposition speed of bone apatite in SBF. As depicted in Fig. 5.12B, the filamentous pseudopodia of osteoblasts grow into the TiO$_2$ nanotubes, effectively increasing the bone growth and osseointegration on the implant's surface. Moreover, the irregularly oriented TiO$_2$ nanotube arrays possess a higher degree of roughness, so the adhesion of bone marrow mesenchymal stem cells significantly increases and thus can rapidly spread, which shows that the rough TiO$_2$ surface has better ability to induce the deposition of osteoblasts [32–35].

5.5 Wear-resistant coatings on TLM alloy

Up to now, the practical surface nanocrystallization of biomedical Ti alloys has mainly focused on the surface self-nanocrystallization caused by surface machining, of which the successful methods include mechanical grinding, ultrasonic shot blasting, and high-speed impact. The surface mechanical attrition treatment (SMAT) and SFT are new surface nanocrystallization technologies that have emerged in the last decade. Their simple operation processes do not cause peeling and separation between the surface nanocrystalline and substrate structures, and they have great application potential, providing ideal conditions for studying grain refinement caused by strong plastic deformation and related mechanical behaviors [36,37]. The surface nanocrystallization of metal materials endows the surface with new surface structure and conditions, which not only maintain or even enhance the mechanical property of materials, but also give the materials the advantages of nanobiology [38].

Numerous studies have shown that, compared to the coarse-grained materials, nanomaterials have more grain boundaries and more active surface hydrophilic characteristics, thereby affecting the interactions between the surface of the artificial prostheses and proteins during the initial stage of implantation. This further has an influence on the functional expression of related genes of osteoblasts on the implant surface, playing an important role in the early healing of the bone-implant interface [38—41]. In addition, the surface hardness, wear resistance, and corrosion resistance of Ti alloys are also improved greatly after SMAT, which can improve the tribological properties of Ti alloy joints and promote the applications of Ti alloy materials in artificial joint prostheses. This section mainly introduces the hard wear-resistance modified layer obtained by SFT on the surface of the novel near β TLM alloy, and analyzes the macroscopic morphology, microstructure, phase composition, surface hardness, and corrosion resistance of the hard surface-modified layer.

5.5.1 Surface hardening modification on TLM alloy

After SFT, along the depth direction of the TLM alloy plates with solid solution state (SSS) has formed three regions roughly: surface area I with indistinguishable grain boundaries, twin area II, and Ti substrate III with no deformation. As depicted in Fig. 5.13, compared to SFT-treated TLM alloy plate with SSS, along the depth direction of the aged TLM alloy plate two obvious regions have formed: surface area I with indistinguishable grain boundaries and substrate area II with no deformation. It is obvious that in the region of the aged TLM alloy surface, no grain boundary distribution can be observed, and there are obvious defects such as gullies, the direction of which is roughly parallel to the alloy surface, suggesting that the main flow direction of the alloy in this area is parallel to the alloy surface. With the increase in depth of the hardening treatment, an obvious cross section emerges between surface area I and nondeformed substrate area II, the grain size abruptly changes at the interface, and it is clear that the grains are stretched out

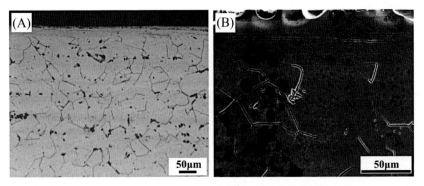

FIGURE 5.13 (A) Morphology of the aged TLM alloy after the SFT treatment. (B) SEM morphology at the interface between the alloy surface and the substrate. *SFT*, sliding friction treatment; *SEM*, scanning electron microscope.

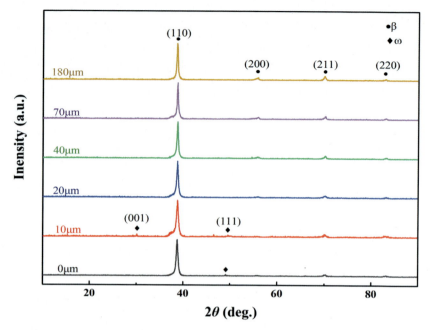

FIGURE 5.14 XRD analysis at different depths of the aged TLM alloy after the SFT treatment. *SFT*, Sliding friction treatment; *XRD*, X-ray diffraction.

at the interface. Fig. 5.14 shows the XRD patterns of the aged TLM alloy at the different depths. It can be seen that the ω phase appears on the alloy surface, but with the depth increasing, the ω phase disappears at the depth of 20 μm. Numerous studies showed that in β Ti alloys, a large amount of plastic deformation induces the transformation of the β phase to ω phase, so the Ti alloy surface can be hardened and toughened.

5.5.2 Surface hardness and corrosion resistance of TLM alloy

Hardness is one of the important indicators to measure the mechanical properties of materials. The hardness of the same materials is affected by many factors, such as work hardening, microscopic grain size, phase transformation, and solute atom. Previous studies showed that the smaller the grain size is, the larger the number or area of grain boundaries that hinder the dislocation slip and thus the higher the hardness. Fig. 5.15 shows the gradient change of microhardness of the TLM alloy along the depth direction. It shows that a gradient nanostructure is obtained on the TLM alloy surface after SFT. The surface hardness is enhanced, and the top surface hardness arises from 260 HV of the

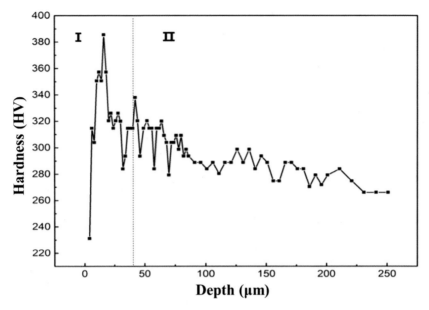

FIGURE 5.15 Microhardness at different depths of the TLM alloy with gradient nanostructures.

original sample to 385 HV, which increases by around 1.5 times. Compared to the change of the gradient structure along the depth direction, the hardness of gradient nanostructure alloy surface decreases fastest from the depth about 20–46 μm. In this area the structures are mainly about 200-nm grains and subgrains, which are formed as a result of the division of the strip structure by the dislocation walls. There are plenty of dislocations in this area. Therefore it can be considered that the hardness improvement in this region results from the combined effect of grain refinement and increase of dislocation density. In the twin region with the depth ranging from 46 to 250 μm, the change rate of hardness was reduced significantly. The grain size in this region was the same as that of the substrate, and the dislocation density in the grain was low. However, there are a large number of twin deliveries and obvious dislocation pileup around the twin boundary, implying that the twins play a major role in strengthening and toughening in this region.

The dynamic potential polarization results of the TLM alloy before and after SFT are depicted in Fig. 5.16. The corrosion current density (i_{corr}) of the TLM alloy with gradient nanograins (NG) is slightly smaller than that of the TLM alloy with primitive coarse grains (CG), while the TLM alloy with NG shows an obviously higher corrosion potential (E_{corr}) than that of TLM alloy with CG. During the anode reaction stage, the corrosion current of the NG alloy is lower than that of the CG alloy

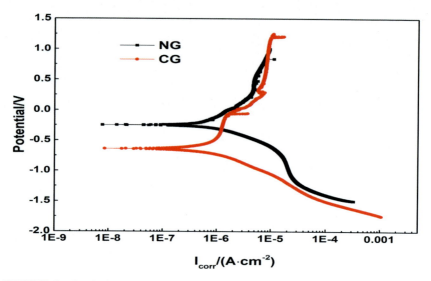

FIGURE 5.16 Electrochemical polarization curves of the TLM alloy before and after SFT. *SFT*, Sliding friction treatment.

at the same voltage, which also suggests that the surface corrosion resistance of the TLM alloy after SFT is obviously improved.

Electrochemical impedance spectroscopy is an effective method of measuring the electrochemical corrosion behaviors of metal electrodes. To further understand the influence of grain size refinement and microstructure change on the electrochemical corrosion behaviors of materials, an electrochemical impedance test of the TLM alloy in 3.5% NaCl solution was conducted. Fig. 5.17 shows the electrochemical impedance spectra of the TLM alloy before and after SFT. The loop of the NG sample at low frequencies is obviously smaller than that of the CG sample. The size of the impedance loop is proportional to the corrosion resistance, further indicating that the electrochemical corrosion resistance of the TLM alloy after surface nanocrystallization hardening treatment is better than that of the original coarse crystal alloy, which is consistent with the above-mentioned results of the dynamic potential polarization tests.

5.6 Anticoagulant coatings on TLM alloy

Improving blood compatibility and reducing the rate of late restenosis are always the focus of efforts to develop better cardiovascular interventional materials. The acceleration of endothelialization *via* the biological decoration and grafting of large molecules (proteins, heparin,

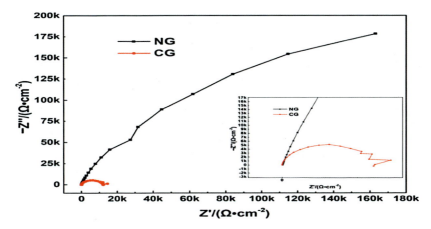

FIGURE 5.17 Electrochemical impedance spectra of the TLM alloy before and after SFT. *SFT*, Sliding friction treatment.

etc.) on the biomedical metal surface are research hotspots. In particular, the selective adsorption and endothelialization on the surface of materials can benefit from the changes of the surface structures and states of materials such as surface morphology, hydrophilicity and hydrophobicity, charge, and surface energy, hence further realizing the biological recognition and treatment. Generally speaking, the smoother surface of vascular stent materials is beneficial for reducing platelet adhesion and thrombus formation, while the negatively charged oxide film on the Ti surface can inhibit thrombus formation and improve blood compatibility and anticoagulation [19].

Surface-modified coatings or films have become among the important ways to effectively improve the anticoagulation of traditional materials and have attract broad attention in the 21st century. To further enhance the blood compatibility of the TLM alloy and endow it with the function of inducing anticoagulant blood, this section mainly introduces the TiO_2 films coated on the TLM alloy *via* the sol–gel method by our research group. After the activation treatment of this film, heparin and albumin were fixed on the surface of the coating by layer-by-layer electrostatic self-assembly. Finally, the changes of anticoagulant properties before and after the surface modification of the TLM alloy were investigated and analyzed.

5.6.1 Preparation and activation of TiO_2 films

The sol–gel method was chosen by our group to prepare the TiO_2 film. Briefly, $Ti(OC_4H_9)$ was used as the sol precursor, glycol methyl ether was used as a solvent, and a small amount of hydrolytic inhibitor ethyl acetoacetate and dry crack inhibitor formamide were added. The film was fabricated by spin coating, put in a vacuum drying oven, slowly heated to 100°C, for the predrying treatment, and then placed in a box-type resistance furnace to heat up to 600°C, where it was held for 1 hour, followed by natural cooling in the furnace to room temperature.

The TLM alloy coated with the TiO_2 film was sequentially treated with a mixed solution of hydrochloric acid and hydrogen peroxide and then a mixed solution of acrylamide and nitric acid to introduce the OH^- and NH_2^- active groups onto the film surface. In the end, the sample was rinsed in 0.05 mol L^{-1} NaOH solution, then washed in hot water and dried.

5.6.2 Self-assembly of heparin and albumin

Biological-grade bovine serum albumin (albumin), heparin, and dextran sulfate were selected. The citric acid solution (1 mg L^{-1}) containing albumin and heparin, phosphate buffer solution (pH = 7.4), and 2.5% glutaraldehyde solution was first prepared, and ten TLM samples coated with the TiO_2 films and activated with functional groups were selected. All samples were immersed in the albumin solution (1 mg L^{-1}) under acidic conditions (pH = 4.8), and the samples were rinsed after 1 hour reaction, followed by immersion in the dextran sulfate solution (1 mg L^{-1}) with adjusted pH for 1 hour, and were then cleaned. The cleaned specimens were immersed in the heparin solution (1 mg L^{-1}) for 1 hour and were then cleaned, followed by immersion in the dextran sulfate solution (1 mg L^{-1}) with adjusted pH for 1 hour and rinsing. These procedures were repeated five times. Afterwards, the samples were immersed in the glutaraldehyde solution for 1 hour, and the obtained samples were finally ultrasonicated in the phosphate buffered saline solution and dried for further incorporation of the heparin-albumin multilayer composite films on the TiO_2 film surface *via* layer-by-layer self-assembly.

5.6.3 Surface characterization of composite coatings

From the SEM images of the surface-modified TLM alloy in Fig. 5.18A and B, it can be seen that a smooth, dense, and flat coating is obtained on the TLM alloy surface *via* the above multistep surface treatment. The coating completely covers the TLM alloy surface, and no peeling or broad cracks are observed. Compared to the sol–gel Ti–O films, the films after surface activation and treatment by heparin and albumin showed greatly reduced microcracks and became smoother and denser. The three-dimensional surface morphology of the composite coating is shown in Fig. 5.18C. The average roughness of the coating was 11.3 μm.

For implants that are in direct contact with blood, when blood comes into contact with the surface of foreign body, the plasma protein adsorption occurs first, and the subsequent results are largely determined by the interaction between the blood and the absorbed protein layer. A surface that is too rough tends to absorb fibrin, and platelets can adhere to the surface adsorbed by the fibrin, thus inducing thrombus formation. Meanwhile, the roughness of the material surface is closely related to the surface energy. When the surface roughness increases, the surface energy of nonpolar components of the material surface significantly goes up, thus inducing the adhesion of fibrin and other clotting tissues on the material surface. The rougher surface causes more contact of metals with blood. The larger surface area leads to a greater probability of thrombosis, since the metal surface promotes coagulation [19].

5.6.4 Characterization of blood compatibility of composite coatings

Table 5.2 presents the hemolysis test results of the TLM alloy before and after surface modification by heparin-albumin composite coatings. It can be seen that after the surface anticoagulation treatment the hemolysis

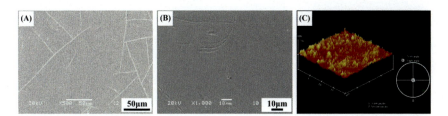

FIGURE 5.18 SEM micrographs of the TiO$_2$ films (A) before and (B) after the heparin-albumin surface decoration. (C) Atomic force microscopy image of the treated TLM. *SEM*, Scanning electron microscope.

TABLE 5.2 Hemolysis rate of the TLM alloy before and after surface modification.

Samples	Absorbance					Average hemolysis rate (%)
	1	2	3	4	5	
Negative control group	0.022	0.021	0.022	0.021	0.021	—
Positive control group	0.923	0.915	0.918	0.920	0.921	—
TLM alloy	0.029	0.028	0.029	0.025	0.027	0.713
Heparinized TLM alloy	0.024	0.027	0.023	0.025	0.026	0.401

rate of the material decreases from 0.713% to 0.401%, far less than 5% of the requirement of implant hemolysis rate stipulated by Chinese national standards. The reason is that the albumin biological layer is formed on the substrate surface after the albumin decoration. The albumin biological layer has better biocompatibility than the bare metals or alloys and does not adsorb fibrin and red blood cells, which reduces the damage to red blood cells in the blood, hence improving the blood compatibility performance of the TLM alloy. In the meantime, after the surface activation treatment the incorporation of the hydrophilic functional groups of −OH and −NH$_2$ on the material surface can improve the hydrophilicity of materials. The hydrophilicity of the material surface is closely related to the blood compatibility of the biomaterials. The hydrophilic surface is conducive to the adhesion and growth of cells, since cell membrane has a certain hydrophilicity, while the hydrophobicity of the material surface is an important cause of hemolysis. For the anticoagulant materials the better hydrophilicity of the material surface corresponds to the smaller interface energy with blood, so the adsorption amount of fibrin and platelets is smaller, meaning better anticoagulant performance [31].

Fig. 5.19 demonstrates that few platelets adhere to the film surface after anticoagulant modification by the heparin-albumin composite

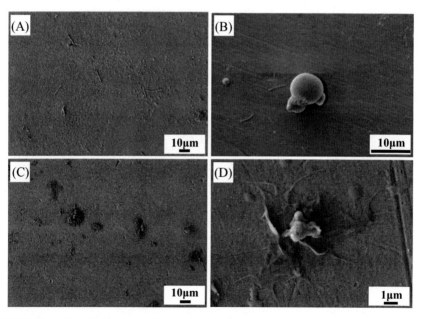

FIGURE 5.19 SEM micrographs of platelet adhesion on the surface of the TLM alloy with and without the heparin-albumin composite films. (A) With treatment. (B) Enlarged image of part A. (C) Without treatment. (D) Enlarged image of part C. *SEM*, Scanning electron microscope.

coatings (Fig. 5.19A), and the attached platelets are integral and show no signs of activation, such as deformation and aggregation (Fig. 5.19B). Fig. 5.19C and D shows that the platelets attached on the surface of the TLM substrate without the anticoagulant treatment are obviously activated and show some pseudopodia, which may cause blood clotting and further formation of subacute thrombosis. This means that the anticoagulant property of the TLM alloy surface can be greatly improved by treatment of the heparin-albumin composite coatings and can meet the requirements of clinical applications.

The coagulation mechanism on the surface of materials is thought to involve complex reactions, in which plasma proteins, coagulation factors, and cells in the blood participate. The reactions become more complicated because of the intervention of materials [41]. The contact of materials with blood result in coagulation and thrombosis, whose major route is the activation of the blood coagulation and cell systems (mainly platelets). For the implants that are in direct contact with blood, the adsorption of plasma proteins occurs first when the blood contacts the surface of a foreign body. However, albumin reduces platelet adhesion [42,43]. Taking advantage of this feature, surface modification is used for the implant materials to make their surface beneficial for the adsorption of ideal proteins. For example, when the amount of albumin reaches a certain proportion and does not cause the denaturation reaction of adsorbed proteins, a good blood-compatible interface is formed, which is an effective way to improve the antithrombotic property of materials. This work makes use of the characteristics of TiO_2 as a n-type semiconductor to suppress the adsorption of fibrinogen on the material surface and then form an albumin precoating on the substrate surface by covalently grafting the active albumin. Under these combined effects, the adsorption and activation of fibrin and platelets on the surface of materials at the initial stage of implantation are prevented, respectively, thus alleviating the exogenous coagulation reaction. Simultaneously, heparin can specifically bind to antithrombin III (AT-III), suppresses thrombin and Xa, and blocks the cascade reactions of endogenous coagulation, which further improves the blood compatibility and anticoagulation properties of the TLM alloy.

5.7 Antimicrobial coatings on TLM alloy

Owing to their excellent biocompatibility, corrosion resistance, and excellent comprehensive biomechanical properties, Ti alloys have gradually become the preferred material for hard tissue substitutes and restorations such as dental implants and artificial joints [44]. However, the surrounding tissue is at risk of infection after implantation of artificial prostheses made of Ti alloys or other materials. The data show that the infection rates of total hip and elbow arthroplasty are 0.1%–1% and 1%–4%, respectively, and the infection rate of metal-to-metal joint prostheses is higher than that of metal-to-polymer prostheses [45]. Once the infection happens and cannot be controlled by conventional antibiotic drugs, it is necessary to remove the implant and perform the operation again, and the patient may even face the risks of amputation and death, which brings great physical and mental pain and economic burden to the patient. Since implants contact human tissues *via* their surfaces, the surface antibacterial property of biomaterials has been drawing attention. Inorganic antibacterial coatings represented by silver-loaded coatings have attracted more and more attention because of their advantages, such as broad-spectrum sterilization, no drug resistance, and low toxic side effects. Comprehensively considering the safety and antibacterial properties, silver ions are the best antibacterial metal ions among various metal ions with antibacterial function that have been found so far. Silver ions have a strong affinity with the enzymes containing the —SH group in the microorganisms and can form irreversible sulfur-silver compounds with the above enzymes at very low concentrations, destroying the activity of microbial cells, causing their death, and destroying the DNA molecules of microorganisms [46,47].

However, the effective content of silver in the current silver-loaded coatings is relatively low, and the silver elements that are physically attached to the surface are released rapidly after implantation, resulting in excessive concentration of antibacterial silver in the early stage, which can have toxic side effects. Furthermore, the antibacterial time is too short, and the clinical treatment effect is poor. This section mainly introduces the preparation of the silver-loaded porous antibacterial coatings using a two-step electrochemical method to endow the TLM alloy with good antibacterial properties. The TiO_2 nanotubes were first prepared by the AO method on the TLM alloy surface as the precoating, followed by the adhesion of silver to the precoating surface *via* physical adsorption, and the samples were eventually treated in electrolyte containing silver by MAO. This provides a novel strategy for the development of silver-loaded antibacterial coatings on Ti alloys.

5.7.1 Preparation and phase characterization of antimicrobial coatings

TLM alloy circular slices (Φ10 mm × 2 mm) and copper sheet were used as the anode and cathode, respectively, and the anode oxidation electrolyte consisted of 0.5% NH_4F, 2% H_2O, and 97.5% ethylene glycol. 60 V DC was applied. After the AO treatment for 4 hours, the samples

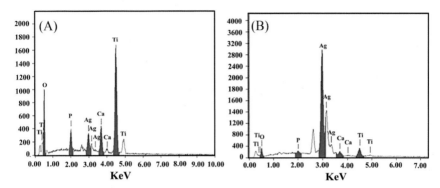

FIGURE 5.20 EDS patterns of (A) the NT-Ag-MAO coatings and (B) nanoparticles on the coating surface. *EDS*, Energy dispersive spectroscopy; *MAO*, microarc oxidation.

were ultrasonically cleaned with deionized water for 30 minutes and dried in vacuum. The samples were then immersed in 1 mol L^{-1} AgNO$_3$ for 2 hours and subsequently irradiated by ultraviolet light with a central wavelength of 253.7 nm for 5 hours. The silver-loaded anodized precoated samples (NT-Ag) were immersed in an electrolyte solution composed of 0.02 mol L^{-1} β-sodium glycerophosphate, 0.16 mol L^{-1} calcium acetate, and 0.2 mol L^{-1} silver for MAO (NT-Ag-MAO). The power supply was kept in constant voltage mode with a voltage of 350 V, a frequency of 100 Hz, and a duty ratio of 40%, and the treatment time was 30 minutes. Finally, the morphology of the prepared samples was observed by SEM, and the composition of the film was detected by energy-dispersive spectroscopy (EDS) attached to SEM.

The EDS spectra of the silver-loaded porous coating are shown in Fig. 5.20. The coating surface contains relatively more Ag as well as Ca, P, Ti, and O. The major elements of the coating are Ti and O with weight percentages of 44.20% and 36.85%, respectively, which mainly come from the TiO$_2$ produced by AO and MAO on the coating surface. The weight percentages of Ca and P are 7.64% and 3.14%, respectively, whereas the weight percentage of the Ag is 8.16%. The micropores in the precoating and secondary MAO coating provide conditions for the abundant fixation of silver on the surface and inside the coating, while the MAO treatment in the silver-containing electrolyte may also further introduce the silver into the surface or inner wall of the coating to obtain silver-loaded coatings with a high content of silver [48].

5.7.2 Characterization of surface morphology of coatings

The AO precoating on the surface of the TLM Ti alloy sample was immersed in the 1 mol L^{-1} AgNO$_3$ solution for 2 hours and irradiated

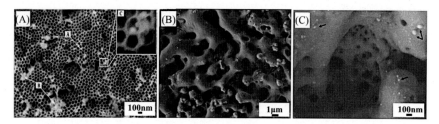

FIGURE 5.21 SEM morphology of (A) the silver-loaded TiO$_2$ nanotube MAO precoating (NT-Ag), (B) the silver-loaded MAO coating (NT-Ag-MAO), and (C) nanoparticles on the coating surface. *SEM*, Scanning electron microscope; *MAO*, microarc oxidation.

by ultraviolet for 5 hours. The macroscopic color of the sample surface gradually darkened and finally appeared black. The surface morphology SEM images are shown in Fig. 5.21A. It can be seen that a large number of dense TiO$_2$ nanotube arrays with an average tube diameter of 123 nm are formed on the surface of the TLM alloy sample after AO. After immersion in AgNO$_3$ and irradiation by ultraviolet light, plenty of fine particles with sizes of 100–500 nm are adsorbed on the surface and inside the nanotube layer. Analysis shows that these particles mainly contain silver, which is also the major reason for the blackening of the precoating surface.

The porous anodized precoating is composed of densely arranged nanotubes and large exposed surfaces, which result in a larger specific surface area and higher surface energy of the nanotube coating and make it easier for the silver salt solution to adhere to the surface to reduce the system energy. After soaking in the silver salt solution, some of the silver salt solution even enters the nanotubes and finally decomposes in the tube. The surface of the sample after further MAO treatment demonstrates a complex and diverse ravine-like shape. The protruding parts of the ravines appear to be molten and rapidly cooled by liquid spray, and the surface is relatively rough and contains a large number of small holes with diameters of less than 1 μm as shown in Fig. 5.21B. It obviously differs from the porous and volcanic crater-like microscopic morphology of samples prepared by common MAO. We believe that it may be the traces left by the previous nanotubes after being melted. This morphology suggests that during the MAO process, the previous precoating is broken down by the arc and the TiO$_2$ nanotubes melt at the high temperature resulted from the MAO [49]. Many silver-containing particles are attached to the surface of the NT-Ag coating. The location and aggregation state of these particles are mainly as follows: attaching to the nanotube orifice in the form of particles; agglomerating together to plug the surface of the nanotube arrays and even large flaky silver-containing particles locally plugging the nanotube orifice; and attaching to the inner wall of the nanotube and even going deeply into the nanotube orifice for a certain distance. EDS point scanning was performed on the particles indicated by the arrows in Fig. 5.21C, and the results confirm that the major element of the bright particles on the coating surface was silver and that the weight percentages of Ag, Ti, O, Ca, and P were 84.01%, 5.24%, 8.09%, 2.10%, and 0.56%, respectively. Hence with the aid of the rough and high-specific-area porous structure of the AO precoating, a better silver-carrying adsorption capacity can be obtained, which is beneficial for the further preparation of coatings with a larger silver-carrying amount by MAO.

Many silver particles are uniformly distributed on the surface of the coating and the inner wall of the hole, as shown in Fig. 5.21C and the arrows shown in the figure. Most of the particles are less than 100 nm in diameter, and a few particles reach hundreds of nanometers in size and appear as molten droplets. Purely physically adsorbed silver will be released quickly in the body fluids in the early postoperative period, resulting in a high concentration of silver ions, which may cause cytotoxicity, the antibacterial ability to decay too quickly in the later stage, and difficulty in achieving stable and sustained release of antibacterial agents and long-term antibacterial effects. In this study, *via* the violent physical and chemical reactions in the MAO process, the embedded micro-sized and nano-size silver particles on the surface, the inner wall of the micropores, and inside of the coating on the TLM alloy were obtained, and they may alleviate this problem [50–53].

5.7.3 Characterization of antimicrobial properties of coatings

To verify the antibacterial abilities of the coatings, the most common strain of *Staphylococcus aureus* (ATCC6538, sixth generation culture) was selected, and experiments were carried out under the conditions of laboratory facilities and safety management regulations in accordance with GB19489. The tests were divided into two groups: the silver-loaded MAO coating (NT-Ag-MAO) group and the nonsilver common MAO coating control group (MAO). The antibacterial abilities were measured by the spread plate method according to GB/T 21866-2008 and GB 4789.2-2010. First, the *S. aureus* solution was dropped onto the surface of the silver-loaded porous coating and silver-free control sample, that is, the silver-free pure Ti surface with the MAO coating. The culture solution was then diluted 1000 times, and the Tween 80 surfactant was added to the solution and uniformly dispersed. Afterwards, the samples were cultured at 37°C in the 95% relative humidity under dark conditions. After incubation for 1, 4, and 7 days, colony counts were performed. To obtain stable and accurate data, three parallel samples labeled samples 1, 2, and 3 were set for each group of data. The average value of colony counts was used to calculate the inhibitory rate (η) according to the following formula:

$$\eta = \frac{D_e - D_n}{D_e}$$

where η is the inhibitory rate, D_e is the number of colonies on the control sample, and D_n is the number of colonies on the testing sample.

To visually verify the antibacterial effect of the coating, a certain amount of the LIVE/DEAD fluorescent staining solution was dripped onto the surface of the samples after inoculation and incubation of the bacteria for 1, 4, and 7 days. This kit contains two kinds of stain solution: SYTO9, which makes live bacteria emit green fluorescence, and PI, which makes dead bacteria emit red fluorescence, clearly distinguishing live bacteria from dead bacteria. After staining and fixing, the sample was observed by an FV1000 laser confocal microscope. The growth of colonies after different culture times and dilutions is shown in Fig. 5.22.

Counting was assisted by the Image J software, and the antibacterial rate of the silver-loaded MAO coating, NT-Ag-MAO, was calculated according to the formula. As shown in Fig. 5.23, the data of the three parallel samples have high consistency. After taking the average value, the antibacterial rates of the silver-loaded coating, NT-Ag-MAO, can

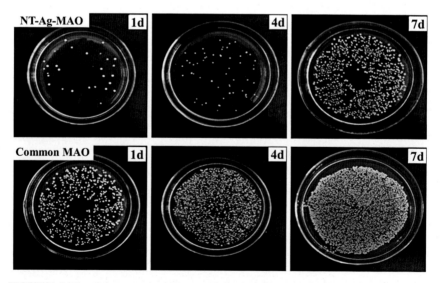

FIGURE 5.22 Colony aggregation on the NT-Ag-MAO coating and common MAO coating after incubation for 1, 4, and 7 days. *MAO*, Microarc oxidation.

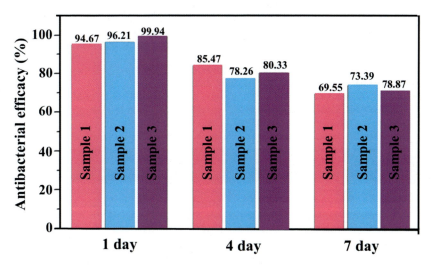

FIGURE 5.23 Antibacterial efficacy of the NT-Ag-MAO coating after incubation for 1, 4, and 7 days. *MAO*, Microarc oxidation.

reach 96.94%, 81.35%, and 71.27% after incubation for 1, 4, and 7 days, respectively. Thus the silver-loaded coating, NT-Ag-MAO, has significantly efficient antibacterial ability compared to the silver-free control sample. Its antibacterial ability weakens over time, which is basically consistent with the release rate of silver ions. It can still kill more than 70% of the total bacteria after 7 days, showing good long-term antibacterial abilities.

References

[1] S. Faghihi, A.P. Zhilyaev, J.A. Szpunar, F. Azari, H. Vali, M. Tabrizian, Nanostructuring of a titanium material by high-pressure torsion improves pre-osteoblast attachment, Advanced Materials 19 (2007) 1069–1073.

[2] D. Kubacka, A. Yamamoto, P. Wieciński, H. Garbacz, Biological behavior of titanium processed by severe plastic deformation, Applied Surface Science 472 (2019) 54–63.

[3] J. Lu, Y. Zhang, W. Huo, W. Zhang, Y. Zhao, Y. Zhang, Electrochemical corrosion characteristics and biocompatibility of nanostructured titanium for implants, Applied Surface Science 434 (2018) 63–72.

[4] W. Huo, L. Zhao, W. Zhang, J. Lu, Y. Zhao, Y. Zhang, *In vitro* corrosion behavior and biocompatibility of nanostructured Ti6Al4V, Materials Science and Engineering: C 92 (2018) 268–279.

[5] Y. Yang, K.-H. Kim, J.L. Ong, A review on calcium phosphate coatings produced using a sputtering process—an alternative to plasma spraying, Biomaterials 26 (2005) 327–337.

[6] A.J. Tonino, B.C. van der Wal, I.C. Heyligers, B. Grimm, Bone remodeling and hydroxyapatite resorption in coated primary hip prostheses, Clinical Orthopaedics and Related Research 467 (2009) 478–484.

[7] C. Capuccini, P. Torricelli, F. Sima, E. Boanini, C. Ristoscu, B. Bracci, et al., Strontium-substituted hydroxyapatite coatings synthesized by pulsed-laser deposition: *in vitro* osteoblast and osteoclast response, Acta Biomaterialia 4 (2008) 1885–1893.

[8] A.M. Pietak, J.W. Reid, M.J. Stott, M. Sayer, Silicon substitution in the calcium phosphate bioceramics, Biomaterials 28 (2007) 4023–4032.

[9] K. Oya, Y. Tanaka, H. Saito, K. Kurashima, K. Nogi, H. Tsutsumi, et al., Calcification by MC3T3-E1 cells on RGD peptide immobilized on titanium through electrodeposited PEG, Biomaterials 30 (2009) 1281–1286.

[10] N. Ohtsu, K. Sato, A. Yanagawa, K. Saito, Y. Imai, T. Kohgo, et al., CaTiO3 coating on Ti for biomaterial application—optimum thickness and tissue response, Journal of Biomedical Materials Research Part A 82 (2007) 304–315.

[11] G. Mendonça, D.B. Mendonça, F.J. Aragao, L.F. Cooper, Advancing dental implant surface technology—from micron-to nanotopography, Biomaterials 29 (2008) 3822–3835.

[12] L. Richert, F. Vetrone, J. Yi, S. Zalzal, J. Wuest, F. Rosei, et al., Surface nanopatterning to control cell growth, Advanced Materials 20 (2008) 1488–1492.

[13] F. Variola, F. Vetrone, L. Richert, P. Jedrzejowski, J. Yi, S. Zalzal, et al., Improving biocompatibility of implantable metals by nanoscale modification of surfaces: an overview of strategies, fabrication methods, and challenges, Small 5 (2009) 996–1006.

[14] B. O'Brien, W. Carroll, The evolution of cardiovascular stent materials and surfaces in response to clinical drivers: a review, Acta Biomaterialia 5 (2009) 945–958.

[15] J. Steffel, F.R. Eberli, T.F. Lüscher, F.C. Tanner, Drug-eluting stents—what should be improved? Annals of Medicine 40 (2008) 242–252.

[16] F. Wen, N. Huang, H. Sun, G. Wan, P.K. Chu, Y. Leng, The study of composition, structure, mechanical properties and platelet adhesion of Ti–O/TiN gradient films prepared by metal plasma immersion ion implantation and deposition, Nuclear Instruments and Methods in Physics Research Section B: Beam Interactions with Materials and Atoms 222 (2004) 81–90.

[17] J. Daemen, P. Serruys, Drug-eluting stent update 2007: part I: a survey of current and future generation drug-eluting stents: meaningful advances or more of the same? Circulation 116 (2007) 316–328.

[18] F.S. Czepluch, J. Waltenberger, Vascular endothelial growth factor protein levels and gene expression in peripheral monocytes after stenting: a randomized comparative study of sirolimus-eluting and bare-metal stents, European Heart Journal 29 (2008) 1924–1925.

[19] Z. Yu, S. Yu, J. Cheng, X. Ma, Development and application of novel biomedical titanium alloy materials, Acta Metallurgica Sinica 53 (2017) 1238–1264.

[20] M.S. Caicedo, R. Desai, K. McAllister, A. Reddy, J.J. Jacobs, N.J. Hallab, Soluble and particulate Co-Cr-Mo alloy implant metals activate the inflammasome danger signaling pathway in human macrophages: a novel mechanism for implant debris reactivity, Journal of Orthopaedic Research 27 (2009) 847–854.

[21] R. Huang, Y. Han, The effect of SMAT-induced grain refinement and dislocations on the corrosion behavior of Ti–25Nb–3Mo–3Zr–2Sn alloy, Materials Science and Engineering: C 33 (2013) 2353–2359.

[22] R. Huang, Y. Han, Structure evolution and thermal stability of SMAT-derived nanograined layer on Ti–25Nb–3Mo–3Zr–2Sn alloy at elevated temperatures, Journal of Alloys and Compounds 554 (2013) 1–11.

[23] F. Barrere, T. Mahmood, K. De Groot, C. Van Blitterswijk, Advanced biomaterials for skeletal tissue regeneration: instructive and smart functions, Materials Science and Engineering: R: Reports 59 (2008) 38–71.

[24] E.M. Hetrick, M.H. Schoenfisch, Reducing implant-related infections: active release strategies, Chemical Society Reviews 35 (2006) 780–789.

[25] K.C. Popat, M. Eltgroth, T.J. LaTempa, C.A. Grimes, T.A. Desai, Titania nanotubes: a novel platform for drug-eluting coatings for medical implants? Small 3 (2007) 1878–1881.
[26] T. Song, M. Yan, M. Qian, The enabling role of dealloying in the creation of specific hierarchical porous metal structures—a review, Corrosion Science 134 (2018) 78–98.
[27] B. Jiang, J. Zhang, H. Shi, Effect of surface morphology of micro-arc oxide film on bonding strength of titanium alloy/epoxy resin, Journal of Nonferrous Metals 14 (2004) 539–542.
[28] Y. Wang, B. Jiang, T. Lei, L. Guo, Y. Cao, Effects of electrical parameters on the microstructure of microarc oxidation ceramic coatings on Ti6Al4V alloy, Journal of Inorganic Materials 18 (2003) 1325–1330.
[29] Q. Huangfu, K. Xu, Y. Han, Character and mechanism of the film by micro-arc oxidation on titanium alloy, Rare Metal Materials and Engineering 32 (2003) 272–275.
[30] Y. Han, S. Hong, K. Xu, Structure and *in vitro* bioactivity of titania-based films by micro-arc oxidation, Surface and Coatings Technology 168 (2003) 249–258.
[31] H. Li, F. Wu, Q. Shao, T. Fu, C. Sun, X. Wu, Superhydrophilic surface modification of medical near β-type titanium alloy TLM, Ti Industry Progress 28 (2011) 23–26.
[32] W. Zhang, Z. Xi, G. Li, Q. Wang, H. Tang, Y. Liu, et al., Highly ordered coaxial bimodal nanotube arrays prepared by self-organizing anodization on Ti alloy, Small 5 (2009) 1742–1746.
[33] G. Li, W. Zhang, J. Han, J. Zhang, X. Kang, Y. Li, Fabrication of TiO_2 nanotube array film on near-β titanium alloy and its effects on osteoblast growth, Rare Metal Materials and Engineering 39 (2010) 1207–1209.
[34] W. Zhang, G. Li, Z. Xi, J. Zhang, H. Tang, Q. Wang, Self-assembled nanoporous titania layers on Ti alloys by anodic oxidation, Rare Metal Materials and Engineering 41 (2012) 356–359.
[35] S. Yu, Z. Yu, J. Han, X. Ma, G. Wang, M.S. Dargusch, Surface bio-modification by TiO_2 film on biomedical titanium alloy, Heat Treatment of Metals 34 (2009) 63–67.
[36] C. Huang, C. Zhao, P. Han, W. Ji, S. Guo, Y. Jiang, et al., Histological and biomechanical evaluation in the interface between nano-surface titanium alloy implants and bone, Journal of Clinical Rehabilitative Tissue Engineering Research 15 (2011) 3867–3870.
[37] Y. Han, H. Zhuang, J. Lu, Deformation-induced ambient temperature α-to-β phase transition and nanocrystallization in (α + β) titanium alloy, Journal of Materials Research 24 (2009) 3439–3445.
[38] W. Huo, L. Zhao, S. Yu, Z. Yu, P. Zhang, Y. Zhang, Significantly enhanced osteoblast response to nano-grained pure tantalum, Scientific Reports 7 (2017) 40868.
[39] R. Huang, H. Zhuang, Y. Han, Second-phase-dependent grain refinement in Ti−25Nb−3Mo−3Zr−2Sn alloy and its enhanced osteoblast response, Materials Science and Engineering: C 35 (2014) 144–152.
[40] R. Huang, S. Lu, Y. Han, Role of grain size in the regulation of osteoblast response to Ti−25Nb−3Mo−3Zr−2Sn alloy, Colloids and Surfaces B 111 (2013) 232–241.
[41] R. Huang, Y. Han, Effect of surface grain refinement of Ti-25Nb-3Mo-3Zr-2Sn alloy on the regulation of osteoblast behavior, Chinese Orthopaedic Journal of Clinical and Basic Research 5 (2013) 28–34.
[42] D.M.D. Ehrenfest, P.G. Coelho, B.-S. Kang, Y.-T. Sul, T. Albrektsson, Classification of osseointegrated implant surfaces: materials, chemistry and topography, Trends in Biotechnology 28 (2010) 198–206.
[43] X. Wang, F. Zhang, C. Li, Z. Zheng, X. Wang, X. Liu, et al., Improvement of blood compatibility of artificial heart valves *via* titanium oxide film coated on low temperature isotropic carbon, Surface and Coatings Technology 128 (2000) 36–42.
[44] N. Huang, P. Yang, Y. Leng, J. Chen, H. Sun, J. Wang, et al., Hemocompatibility of titanium oxide films, Biomaterials 24 (2003) 2177–2187.

[45] Z. Yu, S. Yu, M. Zhang, J. Han, X. Ma, Design, development and application of novel biomedical Ti alloy materials applied in surgical implants, Materials China 29 (2010) 35–51.
[46] W. Song, H. Ryu, S. Hong, Antibacterial properties of Ag (or Pt)-containing calcium phosphate coatings formed by micro-arc oxidation, Journal of Biomedical Materials Research Part A 88 (2009) 246–254.
[47] W. Chen, S. Oh, A. Ong, N. Oh, Y. Liu, H. Courtney, et al., Antibacterial and osteogenic properties of silver-containing hydroxyapatite coatings produced using a sol gel process, Journal of Biomedical Materials Research Part A 82 (2007) 899–906.
[48] P. Kelly, H. Li, K. Whitehead, J. Verran, R. Arnell, I. Iordanova, A study of the antimicrobial and tribological properties of TiN/Ag nanocomposite coatings, Surface and Coatings Technology 204 (2009) 1137–1140.
[49] K. Das, S. Bose, A. Bandyopadhyay, Surface modifications and cell–materials interactions with anodized Ti, Acta Biomaterialia 3 (2007) 573–585.
[50] S. Yu, Z. Yu, G. Wang, J. Han, X. Ma, M. Dargusch, Biocompatibility and osteoconduction of active porous calcium–phosphate films on a novel Ti–3Zr–2Sn–3Mo–25Nb biomedical alloy, Colloids and Surfaces B 85 (2011) 103–115.
[51] S. Yu, Z. Yu, J. Han, M. Zhang, J. Niu, C. Liu, Preparation and osteogenesis of active secondary microporous on the porous Ti3Zr2Sn3Mo25Nb titanium alloy, China Surface Engineering 25 (2013) 101–106.
[52] S. Yu, Z. Yu, J. Han, J. Niu, G. Wang, M.S. Dargusch, Histocompatibility and osteogenic activity of Ti-5Zr-6Mo-15Nb alloy with surface modification by porous TiO_2/HA coating, Heat Treatment of Metals 9 (2010) 31–36.
[53] R. Huang, Y. Han, S. Lu, Enhanced osteoblast functions and bactericidal effect of Ca and Ag dual-ion implanted surface layers on nanograined titanium alloys, Journal of Materials Chemistry B 2 (2014) 4531–4543.

CHAPTER
6

Development and application of TLM alloy for the replacement and repair of surgical implants

6.1 Development and application of traditional Ti implants

Ti and its alloys have been applied in many fields, including aerospace, power generation, automotive, chemical and petrochemical industry, sporting goods, and the medical industry. This is due to their desirable properties, mainly the relatively high specific strength combined with low density, being nonmagnetic, having good weldability, having excellent resistance to corrosion and heat, and so on. Compared to many other biomedical metal materials, Ti alloys possess lower elastic modulus, higher fatigue strength, and better biocompatibility. At present, CP-Ti, Ti6Al4V, and Ti6Al4V ELI Ti alloys are the most widely used, accounting for approximately 70%−80% of total biomedical Ti alloy raw materials, and the application of β-type Ti alloy materials is about 10%−30% in the world [1−3]. Typical implants and orthopedic devices made of Ti alloys fabricated to Chinese standards are listed in Table 6.1.

Some of the main medical devices in which Ti alloys are used can be summarized as follows.

1. Joint repair and replacement devices (hip, knee, ankle, shoulder, elbow, wrist, finger, etc.)

    According to relevant reports, about 100 million patients in the world suffer from inflammation and trauma of knee and hip joints every year, so numerous replacement surgeries are imperative. Bone and joint replacements in the human body are subjected to rotation,

TABLE 6.1 Typical implants and orthopedic devices made of Ti alloys fabricated to Chinese standards.

Product type	Typical products
Joint devices	Femoral stem, joint part of hip, knee, ankle, shoulder
Bone devices	Bone nail, bone plate, bone screw
Spinal devices	Dorsal vertebra, lumbar and spine fixation system
Cardiovascular	Endovascular stent, cardiac valves, pacemaker
Cranial devices	Stencil, mini-bone plate, mini-bone screw
Dental devices	Root, crown, denture, artificial teeth
Surgical tools	Puncture instrument, bone saw, rongeur

bending, compression, muscle contraction, and other functions of the human body. Therefore the implanted biomaterials require high levels of strength and toughness. Compared with ceramics, stainless steel, and some other materials, the elastic modulus of Ti alloys is closer to that of human bones, which is beneficial to decrease stress shielding and the increase service life. CP-Ti can be used for nonload-bearing or small load—bearing body parts, and Ti6Al4V alloy can be used for large loads. On the other hand, porous Ti prostheses have superior biological activity (osseointegration) and excellent biocompatibility, which can improve bone regeneration and repair. These advantages are crucial for clinical applications [4,5].

2. Dental devices and facial repair or replacement implants (dental implant, crown, clasp, dental arch wire, maxillofacial implant, etc.)

The use of Ti metal in dental applications has increased dramatically over the past 20 years, owing to its resisting corrosion and toxicity in tissues, fewer allergic reactions, being nonmagnetic, and having a low elastic modulus and excellent biocompatibility. Besides its conventional use for osseointegrated implants and their systems, Ti and its alloys has been used in the fabrication of prosthetic devices such as crowns, removable prostheses, partial fixed prostheses, and dental implants. Ti alloy is also used in surgery to repair facial damage when artificial parts may be required to replace facial features lost through damage or disease and thus restore the ability of speak or eat and improve the patient's cosmetic appearance [6,7].

Restorative implant dentistry involves the use of dental components above the tissue line. This includes abutments, posts, cylinders, screws, bars, and overdentures. Surgical implant dentistry involves procedures below the tissue line and includes the use of Ti implants. These implants are used to mimic the functionality of a natural tooth root by acting as an anchor as well as to provide features to support a prosthetic connection. The commonly used Ti-based materials for manufacturing dental implants and allied components are CP-Ti Grades 1–4, Ti6Al4V, Ti6Al4V ELI, and Ti6Al7Nb. NiTi alloy, also known as nitinol, is used in orthodontics for brackets and arch wires. It can also be used in pulp cavity therapy, in which nitinol files are used to clean and shape the pulp cavity. Even though the Ti6Al4V alloy is considered to be one of the most favored metallic materials for biomaterial applications, CP-Ti is often preferred over its Ti alloy counterparts for end osseous dental implant applications.

3. Orthopedic trauma and spinal replacement implants (mesh, plate, bone screw and nut, intramedullary nail, spinal internal fixation system-arc-track private lock pedicle orthopedics fixation system, interbody fusion cage, thoracolumbar internal fixation system, etc.)

   The strength of CP-Ti is not enough for load-bearing implants. Ti6Al4V, Ti6Al4V ELI, and Ti6Al7Nb show good balance of mechanical properties but contain V and Al, which have been designated as harmful elements to living tissues. Some β-type Ti alloys with low modulus and nontoxic elements have been developed as surgically implanted biomaterials to reduce the stress-shielding effect that causes a resorption of the bone [8,9].

4. Surgical tools (scalpel, vessel knife, forceps, hemostatic clamp, anastomat, etc.)

   A wide range of surgical tools are made from Ti-based alloys other than stainless steel. One of their merits in this respect is their lightness, which helps to reduce the surgeon's fatigue. These tools are generally anodized to provide a nonreflecting surface, which is essential in microsurgical operations, such as eye surgery. Tools made of Ti-based alloys can be sterilized repeatedly without compromising the edge or the surface quality, corrosion resistance, and strength. Hence there is also no threat to small, sensitive, implanted electronic devices because Ti-based alloys are nonmagnetic [6].

6.2 Design and novel manufacture of Ti implants

Implanted medical devices that are inserted into the human body or natural cavities are intended to remain in the body for at least 30 days. Owing to the wide variety of surgical implants and their different uses, medical devices must undergo rigorous and scientific geometric structure design and mechanical strength calculations before they are approved for use. In 1961 British orthopedic doctor Charnley developed the first low-wear total hip Ti joint and cured a large number of patients with osteoarthritis [10]. In 1971 Branemark discovered the phenomenon of osseointegration and successfully developed a Ti dental implant system [11].

At present, the stem of the artificial hip joint is designed and manufactured mainly with Ti alloy materials, and the key focus for extending the life of the artificial joint is the design of the friction interface. The commonly used friction pairs include metal-to-polymer, ceramic-to-ceramic, ceramic-to-polymer, and metal-to-metal [12]. A performance comparison of different friction pair materials is shown in Table 6.2.

After the early designs and applications of meshed implants and leaf-shaped implants in dentistry, people began to design screw-shaped and column-shaped teeth implant in large quantities. At present, artificial dental implants mainly adopt a two-segment structure. The lower end (also called the implant neck) is implanted in the alveolar bone, acting as an artificial root and attachment. The upper end consists of the abutment, foundation pile, and artificial denture part. This structure requires a smaller base of the implant denture or even does not need a base, which makes the patient feel more comfortable and attractive in comparison with the results of traditional dental implants.

TABLE 6.2 Comparison of different materials used in joint friction pairs.

Material	Friction factor	Wear rate (mm^3/10^6)	Debris and size	Characteristics	Disadvantages
Natural articular cartilage	0.0025–0.015	–	Absorbable	Porous elastic material, composed of water (80%), biological macromolecules, and cartilage cells	Limited self-healing ability
Metal/polymer (CoCrMo/UHMWP)	0.06–0.08	40	Polyethylene 0.1–0.5 μm	Widely used, nontoxic, not easily degraded	Aseptic loosening by wear and tear, short life
Metal/metal (CoCrMo)	0. 22–0.27	0.3–1	Metal 50–100 nm	Good wear resistance, high survival rate	Easy concentration of metal ions, risk of tumors, high friction
Ceramic/ceramic alumina	0.01–0.07	0.1	Alumina 5–90 nm	Smallest friction, longest life, high requirements for the implanted position	Fragile femoral head, prone to high-frequency abnormal noise

At present, a large number of conventional medical device, such as artificial joints, spinal internal fixation systems, dental implants, bone plates, and bone nails, are usually processed by machining methods. The stem of the artificial joint can also be made into a near net shape through hot die forging, precision casting, and so on, followed by secondary precision machining and postprocessing. Surface processing is also one of the key factors to ensure the performance and quality of medical device products. In the late 1990s, Klüber Technology Company (Germany) produced porous Ti alloy femoral stems by using directional solidification technology, which could biologically induce the ingrowth of bone cells and promote osseointegration, hence avoiding the disadvantages of loosening, sinking, and dislocation caused by cement-aided fixation. Exactech, Zimmer, and Taiwan Union Company made use of Ti microsphere beads or powder at the proximal end of the stem by sintering or plasma spraying. This design further reduces the difference between the elastic modulus of the implantation material and that of bone and is even conducive to bone cell growth and nutrient delivery. In recent years, joint product manufacturers at home and abroad have generally adopted plasma spraying, vacuum plasma spraying, and other technologies to prepare hydroxyapatite (HA) active coating on the proximal end of the joint stem. This is because human bone is a natural composite material composed of osteogenic fiber tissue and HA, and there is better bonding between them.

In view of the obvious biological and mechanical compatibility of porous Ti alloys with bone tissue, researchers in various countries have actively developed advanced preparation technologies for porous medical Ti alloy, which have been widely used, as shown in Table 6.3 [13].

The overall performance of porous Ti implant is greatly improved mainly in the following three aspects:

1. Compared with dense materials, the density, strength, and elastic modulus of porous Ti and its alloys can match the mechanical properties of the replaced bone tissue by adjusting the porosity, which can effectively reduce or eliminate stress shielding. In addition, there is a longer stress platform after elastic deformation in the stress—strain curve of porous Ti alloys; hence they can buffer, absorb shock, and resist impact from external sources, which has considerable significance in the applications for the body's load-bearing parts [14].
2. The unique porous structure and rough inner and outer surfaces of porous Ti materials will facilitate the adhesion, proliferation, and differentiation of human cells; promote the growth of new bone tissue into the pores; and make it easy to form biological fixation between the implant and the bone.

TABLE 6.3 Preparation methods and characteristics of porous titanium alloy.

Preparation methods	Characteristics
Loose sintering	Simple and quick processing. The size and shape of the holes are controlled by that of Ti powder. The holes is highly aspherical, and cracks may be initiated from here under fatigue conditions
Add pore former	Complicated processing and high cost. Big porosity and good osteoinductivity, but the microporous characteristics are difficult to accurately control. The mechanical properties cannot be well matched with the bone tissue.
Organic foam impregnation	Complicated processing, higher porosity rate, good pore connectivity, and no small pore distribution on the pore wall. The mechanical properties cannot be well matched with the bone tissue.
Solid foaming method	Complicated processing, poor pore connectivity. The shape, size, connectivity, and volume percentage of porous Ti deviate with the original powder preform. The requirements of equipment are higher. and the porosity rarely exceeds 50%.
Self-propagating high-temperature sintering	High-purity porous Ti alloy can be obtained with anisotropic pore structure, but the requirements of the equipment are higher.
Titanium fiber sintering method	Titanium fiber mesh implants have excellent biocompatibility, corrosion resistance, load-bearing, and osteoinductive properties *in vivo*.
Slurry foaming	Simple and quick processing. Low cost, good pore connectivity. The porosity can be adjusted. There are small holes on the pore walls, and the process is unstable.
Additive manufacturing	The micropore characteristics and porosity can be adjusted. The three-dimensional shape and microstructure can be personalized with higher efficiency. Special equipment and proprietary raw materials are required.

3. The porous Ti material has unique three-dimensional (3D) interconnected pores, which allow body fluids and nutrients to transmit, promote tissue regeneration and reconstruction, accelerate the healing process, and improve the quality of osseointegration.

Compared with traditional mechanical subtraction technologies, such as turning, milling, planing, and grinding, if additive manufacturing technology is used in the processing of Ti alloy medical devices, it will not only bring greater freedom for design and manufacturing, but also show incomparable advantages in processing cost and efficiency, especially for products with complex structures and individual characteristics. It is also easy to introduce porous intercommunicating structures to increase the biocompatibility of the implants. In particular, 3D printing technology allows the use of different materials and structures in different parts according to the actual application environment or design to give it specific physical and chemical properties in specific areas, which is difficult to achieve with traditional processing methods such as powder sintering.

3D printing technology can perform precise processing of complex parts, which fits the customization requirements of medical devices. Selective laser melting (SLM) is a commonly used 3D printing technology the main principle of which is to use high-intensity laser as the energy source to directly melt the metal powder at high temperature and then deposit it layer by layer. Generally speaking, the components with complex geometric structures manufactured by SLM have high dimensional accuracy and good surface integrity and do not require subsequent complex processing. Because the variability of human bones and the randomness of the morphology of lesions and defects, standardized implants often cannot meet the clinical requirements of patients. Customized products have become the current key development direction for high-end medical device design, manufacturing, and application promotion [15]. Taking the bone plate as an example, the preparation process for a customized rapid prototyping of a Ti alloy device is shown in Fig. 6.1.

Our research group has tested the mechanical properties of porous Ti plates and found that the quasistatic compressive stress–strain curve

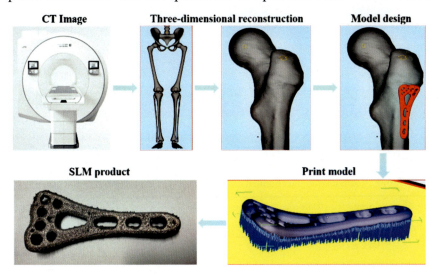

FIGURE 6.1 Schematic diagram of customized rapid prototyping preparation of Ti bone plates.

shows the typical characteristics of porous materials: linear elastic stage, plateau zone, and densification. The plateau stage is a typical feature for highly porous Ti materials, while the low-porosity Ti (≤35%) will appear to have a pseudo-platform, and the slope of the pseudo-platform stage depends significantly on the porosity. As the porosity increases, the slope of the curve in the pseudo-platform stage gradually decreases. The elastic modulus of porous Ti is roughly distributed in the range of 1–18 GPa, the yield strength is approximately distributed in the range of 50–800 MPa, and the compressive strength is in the range of 100–1600 MPa, which can meet the requirements of cortical bone for the elastic modulus. Our research also found that the elastic modulus and strength of porous Ti continue to decrease with increase in porosity. The porous Ti samples with different pore structure parameters and the relationship between elastic modulus, strength, and porosity are shown in Fig. 6.2 and Table 6.4.

In addition, we have successfully fabricated Ti alloy implants with different topologies by using 3D printing technology, as shown in Fig. 6.3.

6.3 Implants for orthopedics and trauma repair

Orthopedic trauma repair devices are passive surgical implants that provide mechanical support for bone, cartilage, tendon, or

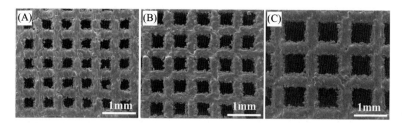

FIGURE 6.2 The porous structure of pure Ti samples produced by laser printing. (A) 400 μm. (B) 500 μm. (C) 600 μm.

TABLE 6.4 Compressive mechanical properties of 3D-printed porous CP-Ti samples.

Pore diameter (μm)		Hole edge thickness (μm)		Porosity (%)		R_p (MPa)	E (GPa)
Designed	Measured	Designed	Measured	Designed	Measured		
400	361.2 ± 11.5	200	239.2 ± 9.9	72.5	69.2 ± 0.8	≈160	≈11
500	451.6 ± 15.1	200	241.8 ± 11.3	78.6	74.1 ± 0.5	≈130	≈9
600	548.2 ± 14.7	200	240.8 ± 2.5	82.9	78.2 ± 0.5	≈90	≈7

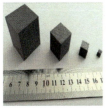 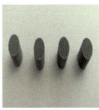 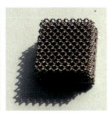 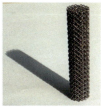

FIGURE 6.3 Ti6Al4V alloy implants with different three-dimensional topologies. *Source: data from L. Luo, S. Yu. Z. Yu, C. Liu, J. Han, J. Niu, Research progress of 3D printing for titanium medical devices, Titanium Industry Progress 32 (2015) 1–5.*

ligament structures, which are mainly used to treat fractures, traumas, defects, and orthopedics [16]. Typical orthopedic trauma repair devices include bone plates, intramedullary nails, bone screws, orthopedic nails, orthopedic rods, femoral neck fixation nails, fracture-binding bands, and orthopedic wires. Ti bone plates are the most widely used for orthopedic trauma repair devices. The following discussion briefly introduces our team's design and development progress on Ti alloy bone plates.

6.3.1 Design of bone plates

To ensure the best possible fit between the bone plate and the human bone, the forging process of the Ti alloy slab is very important. First, it is necessary to obtain the forming condition of the workpiece through simulation calculation to determine the temperature change of the workpiece and the mold, the residual stress of the workpiece, the springback deformation, the mold stress distribution, and the defects. The details are as follows.

1. Five processes are simulated, including heat exchange with the air and the die, deformation, pressure holding and springback.
2. The calculation and simulation results should include mold temperature change, stress distribution in the die, temperature change in the workpiece, metal flow, stress and strain distribution in the workpiece, elastic deformation, and residual stress distribution after springback. The following information is required.
   a. Is the loading speed appropriate?
   b. Analysis of metal fluidity
   c. Temperature distribution, stress, and strain in the bone plate
   d. Damage (crack)
   e. Residual stress, springback, optimization of initial workpiece shape, and initial positioning position.

172   6. Development and application of TLM alloy

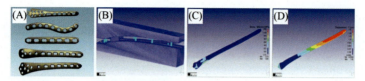

FIGURE 6.4 The simulation pictures of hot forging of Ti alloy bone plates. (A) Bone plates. (B) Forging. (C) Stress. (D) Strain.

The simulation results of hot forging of Ti alloy bone plates are shown in Fig. 6.4.

6.3.2 Processing and pretreatment for the forging of bone plates

1. The specific processing
    a. The first stage: The heat exchange duration between workpiece and the air from the workpiece being taken out from the furnace and put on the mold is about 8 seconds.
    b. The second stage: The heat exchange duration between the workpiece and the bottom die before the workpiece contacting the upper die is about 3 seconds.
    c. The third stage: The forming process, that is, slow deformation of the workpiece until the equipment force reaches 180 t and then stopping when the maximum load force of the half-loaded simulated model is 90 t.
    d. The fourth stage: Pressure holding process; the pressure holding time is 8 seconds.
    e. The fifth stage: The process that the upper mold is lifted and the workpiece rebounds.
2. Setting of the preprocessing parameters for simulation
    a. The blank: Ti6Al4V alloy as annealed, finite element modeling (FEM) grid of tetrahedron with 78,000 pieces, the initial forging temperature at 700°C.
    b. Forging die: Cr12 steel material, 20°C at initial temperature, 45.5 mm s^{-1} in pressing speed, FEM grid 332,000 pieces for the upper and bottom die.
    c. Contact boundary: 0.5 set for the shear friction coefficient between the blank and the die (without lubrication), 11 for heat transfer coefficient (default value of the software).

6.3.3 Hot forging simulation

It can be seen from Fig. 6.5 that when the equipment reaches the set maximum force of 180 T, the Ti workpiece is incompletely in contact with the

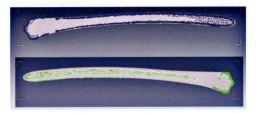

FIGURE 6.5 Contact analysis between Ti workpiece and die at maximum pressure.

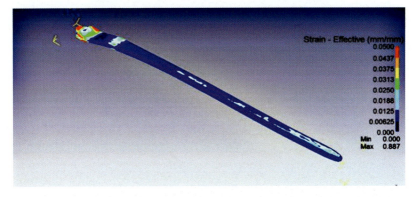

FIGURE 6.6 The overall strain distribution in Ti workpiece at the end of the third stage.

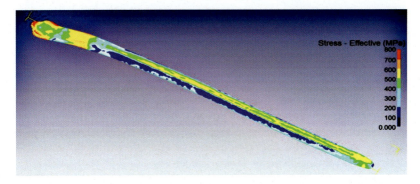

FIGURE 6.7 Equivalent stress distribution in the workpiece at the end of forging.

die (has not been filled). Fig. 6.6 shows the overall strain distribution in the workpiece, from which it can be seen the workpiece can be bent only when the load increase to 180 t, but the workpiece thickness stays nearly constant.

Fig. 6.7 shows that the equivalent stress distribution in the workpiece is largest when the load reaches the maximum in the third stage. Fig. 6.8 shows that in the pressure holding stage, the stress is released to a certain extent while the shape and size of the workpiece are

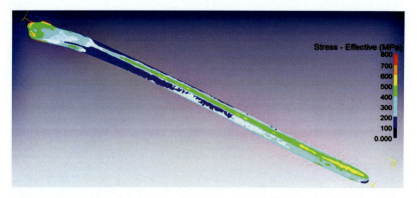

FIGURE 6.8 Equivalent stress distribution in the workpiece at the end of pressure holding.

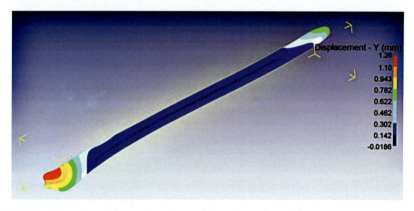

FIGURE 6.9 *Y*-direction rebound deformation of the titanium workpiece.

maintained. Fig. 6.9 shows the size of the rebound deformation of the Ti workpiece along the *Y*-direction. Fig. 6.10 shows the distribution of the equivalent stress before the rebound and the distribution of residual stress after the rebound of the Ti workpiece.

By referring to the finite element numerical simulation analysis results of the processing of the Ti6Al4V alloy bone plate, we have successfully produced a variety of TLM alloy bone plate samples and intramedullary nails, as shown in Fig. 6.11.

6.4 Implants for joint repair and replacement

Artificial hip joints are used mainly for middle-aged and elderly patients with rheumatoid osteoarthritis, femoral head necrosis, and

6.4 Implants for joint repair and replacement   175

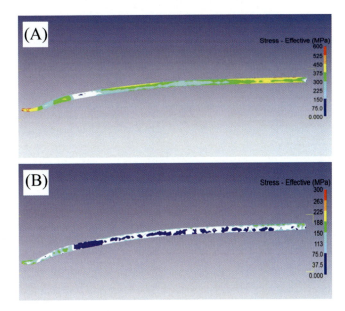

FIGURE 6.10 Stress distribution of the Ti workpiece. (A) Before rebound. (B) After rebound.

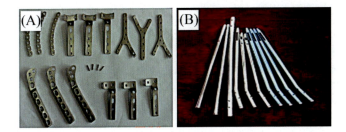

FIGURE 6.11 Some typical samples of TLM alloy. (A) Bone plates. (B) Intramedullary nails.

other serious joint diseases. The main purpose of artificial hip joints is to relieve joint pain, correct deformities, and restore and improve joint movement functions. At present, the artificial joint stem (shank) is generally produced with die forging, precision casting, and other near-net forming processes and then machined with precision computer numerical control (CNC). However, for some patients, about 10 years after the operation, the joint prosthesis suffers service failure. For example, about 90% of Ti6Al4V joint prostheses require secondary surgery within 8–10 years, mainly because of the loosening, sinking, or breaking of the prosthesis resulting from poor biomechanical matching between the

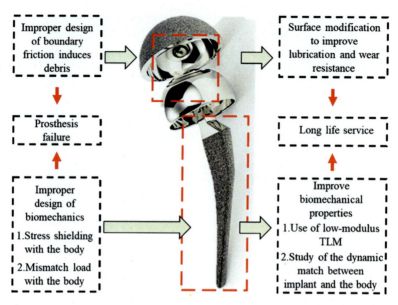

FIGURE 6.12 Schematic diagram of common failure factors and our proposed solutions for hip prostheses.

implants and the surrounding bone tissue, which accounts for 80% of all revision operations [17]. Therefore it is necessary to develop new high-strength and low-modulus medical β-type Ti alloy artificial joints as well as new surface modification technologies. Fig. 6.12 is a schematic diagram of the influencing factors that may cause failure when an artificial hip joint is in service, along with our proposed solutions.

Because of the design of artificial hip joint prostheses, the stress distribution in the femur bone is directly related to prosthesis loosening, sinking, and bone resorption. The early micromovement of the femoral stem and the sinking after bone resorption are the main reasons for the failure of the hip joint. For this, we have carried out research and development on the design and processing of a TLM alloy hip joint femoral stem.

6.4.1 Design of a TLM femoral stem

The design of the femoral stem of the artificial hip joint is shown in Fig. 6.13A. Its key structure and profile include the femoral stem prosthesis (1), the three-sided semicircular cross-sectional groove (2), the oblique groove in the central area (3), the tapered and arc cross-sectional shape at the distal end (4), the circular shape in the middle cross section (5), and the quadratic curve profile for the outer longitudinal section at the distal stem (6). The joint design is not easy to sink or loosen and helps to prolong

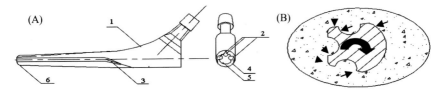

FIGURE 6.13 Schematic diagram for the femoral stem of an artificial hip joint.

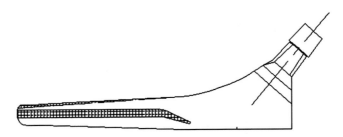

FIGURE 6.14 Schematic diagram of the increase in contact area with the femur by the grooved profile.

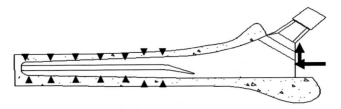

FIGURE 6.15 Schematic diagram of relief of stress concentration by the cone and variable cross-sectional structure.

the life of the prosthesis and to reduce the pain. To fix the femoral stem firmly in the femoral medullary cavity after implantation, that is, without loosening resulting from the torsion and resorption due to the stress shielding of the femoral stem, the longitudinal section at the distal end of the stem is designed as a quadratic curve. The semicircular cross-sectional groove can increase the torsion resistance of the joint, as shown in Fig. 6.13B. This design can increase the contact area with the femur, as shown in Fig. 6.14, which can also relieve the stress concentration and improve the flow of the blood supply to the proximal coating, thus promoting the early formation of osseointegration. The cone structure can effectively disperse the compressive stress on the femur transmitting from the femoral stem, as shown in Fig. 6.15.

6.4.2 Mechanical simulation of the designed hip joint prosthesis

Analysis software can be used for static 3D finite element analysis of stress (strain) distribution in the hip joint prosthesis and to analyze the influence of the material's elastic modulus, Poisson's ratio, and friction pair structure. Through comprehensive analysis of the normal stress, shear stress, and resultant force on the prosthesis, we put forward a new scheme for the design of the prosthesis: the composite friction pair structure HMWPE (the outer, with low modulus and large Poisson's ratio) matching with TLM (the inner, with high strength and low modulus). The radius ratio of the composite structure should be maximized. The finite element simulation results are shown in Figs. 6.16—6.18.

From the perspective of the calculation the larger stress is basically concentrated at the lower half of the prosthesis and the stem-neck junction, and the largest stress appears in the lower half of the prosthesis. Therefore it is necessary to fully consider the force of the lower half of the prosthesis and the environment after implantation. The reduced cross-sectional area

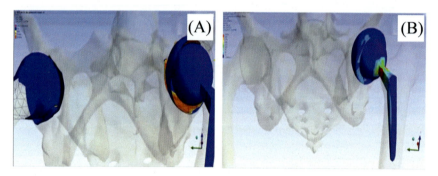

FIGURE 6.16 (A) Deformation and (B) stress in the hip joint prosthesis.

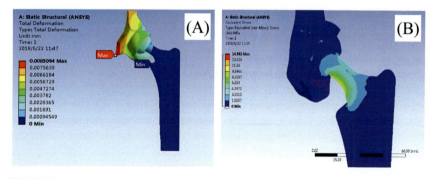

FIGURE 6.17 Total deformation in the hip joint prosthesis in a normal gait.

6.4 Implants for joint repair and replacement

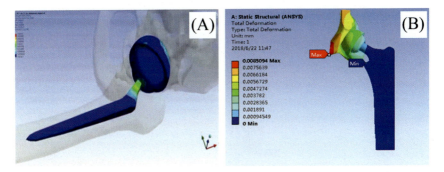

FIGURE 6.18 Simulation analysis of hip joint prosthesis. (A) Stress. (B) Strain.

TABLE 6.5 Specifications of a TLM hip joint prosthesis.

Codes	Neck shaft angle (degree)	Distal diameter, D (mm)	Stem length, L (mm)
A-x-y	135	8, 9, 10, 11, 12, 13, 14, 15	130, 135, 140, 145, 150, 160
B-x-y	131	8, 9, 10, 11, 12, 13, 14, 15	130, 135, 140, 145, 150, 160, 170, 190, 210

Note: A, Angle; x, diameter; y, stem length.

at the stem-neck junction causes the stress to be concentrated there, in which there is a complicated force, so the stem-neck junction is a key part in the prosthesis design. This conclusion came from a simplified bone model, which is not exactly equivalent to a real human femur. It still requires further and more accurate 3D finite element analysis and real biomechanical experiment to verify. Table 6.5 shows the specifications of our preliminary design of a TLM alloy artificial hip joint prosthesis. Fig. 6.19 shows the assembly and exploded view of this design.

6.4.3 Dynamic mechanical simulation and biotribological analysis of the designed hip joint prosthesis

1. Fatigue analysis

    Fatigue test is the key index for evaluating the design of an artificial joint. The fatigue test for traditional artificial hip joints has the characteristics of low cycle frequency (<5 Hz) and a large number of cycles (>5 million). Since the test cycle is long, a large number of samples are required for one test, and multiple devices

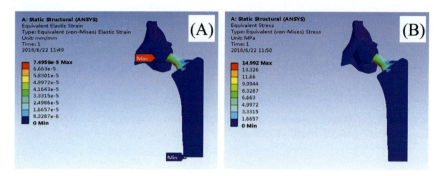

FIGURE 6.19 Assembly and exploded view of artificial joint.

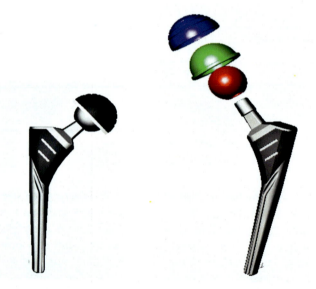

FIGURE 6.20 Simulation analysis of TLM alloy hip joint. (A) Fatigue life. (B) Fatigue damage.

must be tested simultaneously, the test requirements restrict the rapid development and innovation of artificial joint products.

Finite element simulation analysis is a simple, efficient method of quickly evaluating the fatigue performance of an artificial joint. It is based on linear statistical analysis, using existing fatigue analysis software. In the high cycle fatigue simulation analysis of a TLM alloy artificial hip joint, we chose the data of elastic modulus E, Poisson's ratio u, tensile strength R_m, and S—N curve to carry out a static simulation analysis. Fatigue analysis on this basis was then performed. Fig. 6.20 is a simulation analysis of fatigue life and

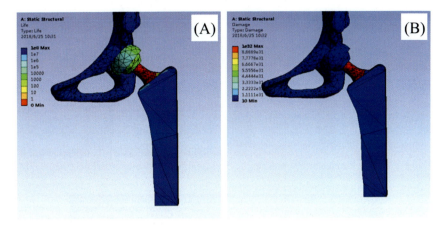

FIGURE 6.21 Cross-sectional analysis of a TLM alloy hip joint. (A) Fatigue life. (B and C) Fatigue damage.

fatigue damage of a TLM alloy hip joint. Fig. 6.21 is the simulation analysis of fatigue life and fatigue damage of a TLM alloy hip joint at its cross section.

The simulation results show that when the maximum cycle number of the TLM alloy stem is 1×10^8, the lateral displacement of the joint head is 0.467–0.545 mm, and the maximum tensile stress of the prosthesis is 15 MPa (at the junction of the joint head and stem). It is very difficult to perform accurate FEM fatigue analysis of the joint prosthesis, but the analysis results are instructive in terms of trends.

2. Biomechanical CAE analysis

When the femoral stem of an artificial hip joint bears the pressure transmitted from the femoral head, the shape of its distal fillet will affect the stress transmission. It is necessary to conduct a biomechanical CAE analysis for this. For the shape design of the distal fillet, the model and finite element meshing of the stem and femur are shown in Fig. 6.22. The stress from the femoral ball head can be decomposed into stress parallel and perpendicular to the axis of the femoral stem. All surfaces of the femoral model are fixed without displacement. The stress distribution cloud diagram for three design conditions of the distal fillet is shown in Fig. 6.23. Fig. 6.24 shows the comparison of the maximum stress values in three conditions.

It can be seen from Fig. 6.23 that the maximum stress in the bone near the distal end of the prosthesis is located at the part, in which the femur contacts with the filleted corner. Fig. 6.23 also shows that when the fillet distal corner of the joint prosthesis transits to a

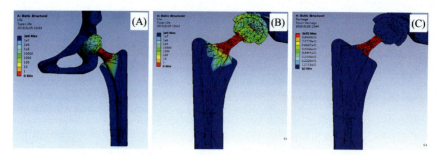

FIGURE 6.22 Finite element meshing for the stem and femur of an artificial hip joint.

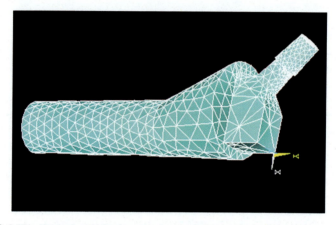

FIGURE 6.23 Diagram of the transition shape of the corner and the stress distribution cloud for different corners of the femur stem. (A) R5 in corner radius. (B) R3 in corner radius. (C) Transition parabola.

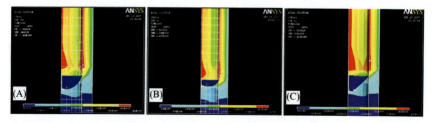

FIGURE 6.24 The transition shape of the distal corner of the prosthesis and the maximum stress for different corners of the femur stem.

parabola profile, the stress on the femur is smallest under the condition of the same lateral displacement of the joint ball head, which indicates that this parabola profile can effectively reduce stress in the femur, thereby reducing the patient's thigh pain resulting from stress.

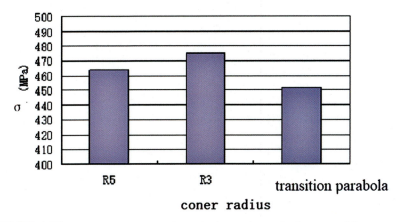

FIGURE 6.25 Schematic diagram of a multiple test device for fatigue and friction.

3. Biotribology analysis

To monitor the variation and their effects on the mechanical parameters of prosthesis materials, friction pair materials, and their interfaces in various and concerned areas in real time, our group independently developed a novel multiple test device for metal fatigue and friction performance, as shown in Fig. 6.25, and we have applied for a Chinese invention patent [18]. The device can be used to study the biomechanical behavior of stress (strain) on the implant and the body bone under long-term service or load conditions as well as the wear morphology and the amount, shape, and size of wear debris produced by the biological friction interface between an implant and bone tissue. By further combining with studies such as the biomechanical behavior of trabecular bone, the micromechanism on joint wear and fatigue damage can be taken, which is also helpful in studying the failure rules in the later stages of artificial joint prosthesis [19,20].

6.4.4 Manufacture process of a TLM femoral stem

The processing route of the TLM femoral stem is as follows:

Raw material (TLM bar, Φ24–30 mm) → Blanking → Turning outer surface → Hot forging → Removing flash and burrs → Removing oxide crusts → Turning → Milling → Wire cutting → Surface treatment → Polishing → Marking

According to the model of the prosthesis, the corresponded diameter bar is selected and cut to the chosen length. An electric furnace is used for heating, and the furnace chamber must be cleaned before charging so that

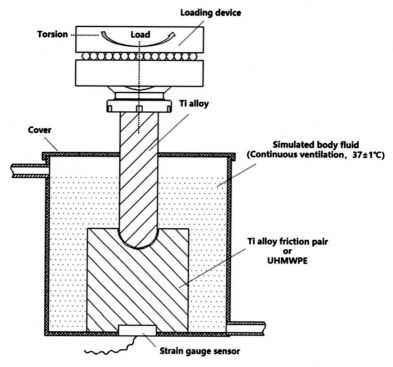

FIGURE 6.26 Forging die and the samples of a TLM hip joint stem.

contaminants such as iron and copper oxide are not present. Forging is carried out on a 20-t friction press. Before forging, the bar blank needs to be sprayed with glass lubricant, and brush engine oil and graphite must be brushed evenly into the upper and lower cavities of the die. After the furnace has been heated to 750°C–950°C, the bar can be put into it. After holding for 0.5 hour, the furnace temperature is gradually raised to 950°C–1050°C, where it is kept for a certain time (depending on the size of the blank). Then the forged femoral stem must undergo solid solution treatment and aging heat treatment, which are carried out in an electric heating furnace. When the furnace temperature rises to 600°C–700°C, the hot mold-forging is loaded into the furnace, kept there for 1–4 hours, and then taken out and air-cooled to room temperature. Fig. 6.26 shows the forging die and forged TLM hip joint stem.

After the forging, the flash and burrs are removed with a grinding wheel. The oxide layer is removed by grinding or sandblasting. The wedge of the distal end and the ball head are treated with precise turning. The grooves and planes are treated by milling. The parabolic part is treated with wire cutting. The whole hip stem is ground and polished. Some typical TLM joint stem samples processed by our research group are shown in Fig. 6.27.

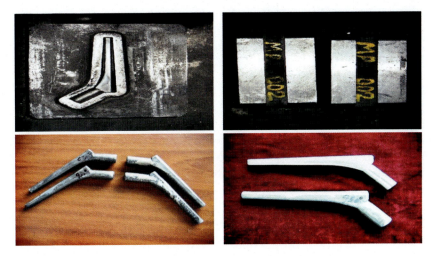

FIGURE 6.27 Some TLM joint samples. (A) Hip joint. (B) Spine joint.

6.5 Implants for oral and maxillofacial repair and replacement of TLM alloy

Artificial dental implants are classified as one-piece or two-section types according to the structure. They are classified as cylinder, threaded cylinder, or composite heteromorphic implants according to the shape. They are also classified as inner join or outer join according to their connection modes. The placement, connection strength, and antirotation of the implants are determined by different connection modes, which have further effects on the stability of the prosthesis. The more suitable the interface of the implants, the lower the potential that micromotion of the interface will happen, which is conductive to maintain the abilities of early loading and the long-term service. The antirotation design of the interface of the implants usually includes internal and external polygonal structure, spline structure, Morse Taper, and so on [21].

The commonly used Ti dental implants have the following problems in clinical application: (1) The elastic modulus of medical Ti alloys such as TC4 and TA2 (widely used worldwide at present) mismatches with that of the bone. (2) The structure design of implants gives rise to stress concentration inevitably and difficulty in processing. (3) There exists some phenomenon like low bonding strength and tending to peel off between the coating of the implants and the substrate. TLM alloy not only possess higher-strength, lower modulus, and higher fatigue limitation, but also has excellent performance of cold and hot processing formability, which makes it suitable for dental implants and other dental devices. Based on a large number of 3D anatomical data and 3D finite element mechanical analysis of teeth and alveolar bone [22], the structural design of the new dental implant mainly includes self-tapping thread, tooth root, spiral edge, hexagonal guiding thread, and fastening thread.

6.5.1 The structural design of a TLM dental implant

The design concepts of the new dental implants include the following: (1) Large pitch grooves are arranged evenly on the circumference of the roots to prevent rotation and reduce the amount of bone excision. (2) The neck of the center screw is treated with Morse taper and thread to reduce the chance of the center screw falling off. (3) The thread is trapezoidal to disperse the root stress effectively. (4) The thickness of the neck is decreased at the gingival area to form a stress relief ring.

1. Antirotation groove design of a TLM dental implant
   The implant may be subjected to reverse rotation force during service, which will loosen the implant and eventually lead to its failure. According to the shape and position of the antispinning groove, several designs are used, as shown in Fig. 6.28. The structure in Fig. 6.28E can effectively prevent reverse rotation and reduce the amount of bone excision during implantation.
2. The thread shape design of a TLM dental implant
   The screw shapes and pitches have a great influence on stress distribution in implants. As shown in Fig. 6.29, compared with the V-shaped design, the thread shape of the nonextrusion state (no initial stress at the interface), such as the rectangular and serrated thread designs, can reduce vertical fretting and make the implant more stable. By comparison the trapezoidal thread shown in Fig. 6.29B is more conducive to the uniform distribution of stress and the fatigue resistance of the implant.

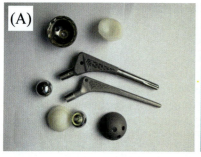 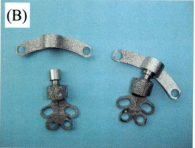

FIGURE 6.28 The design of antirotation grooves. (A) Vertical slot. (B) Neck grooving. (C) Semicircular vertical slot. (D) Spiral groove. (E) Large pitch circular uniform distribution groove.

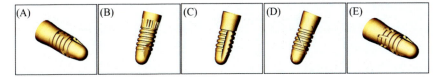

FIGURE 6.29 The shapes designing of the thread. (A) Semicircle. (B) Trapezoid. (C) Triangle. (D) Rectangle. (E) Flat up and tilt below. (F) Tilt up and flat below.

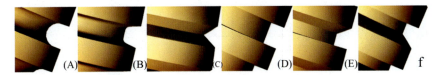

FIGURE 6.30 Thread shape design of a TLM dental implant.

The thread pitch with a vertex angle of 15–30 degrees and 2–3 times the size of an ordinary external thread is more suitable for the biomechanical properties of cancellous bone, as shown in Fig. 6.30. Maintaining a certain width at the screw top is beneficial to reduce osteonecrosis caused by stress concentration. Maintaining a certain height is also beneficial for bone ingrowth and increasing the binding force.

3. The root shape design of a TLM dental implant

    The root shapes of dental implants have a significant effect on the stress distribution in the surrounding bone. A small curvature or geometric discontinuity (stepped) on the implant surface produces much higher stress in the bone than that of a smooth one (cylindrical, cone). In addition, the lower end of it has a certain taper, which is helpful for the self-tapping. The hemispherical shape of the distal end can effectively reduce the stress concentration. The larger diameter of the neck is conducive to dispersing the stress in a larger range. After the above-mentioned analysis we finally chose the root shape shown in Fig. 6.31D, in which the implant is cylindrical in shape.

4. Antirotation pad or coat on the central screw of a TLM dental implant

    We designed the structures such as adding antirotation pads between the center screw and its contact cone of the foundation post, adding antirotation pads to the column part, adding double-threaded antirotation structure, or preparing antistripping coating on the threaded part. Finally, the structure of the central screw with antirotation coating was adopted through experiments and analysis; the result is shown in Fig. 6.32D.

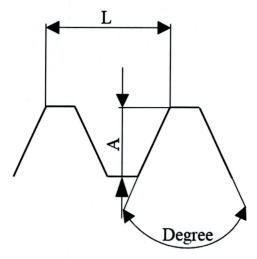

FIGURE 6.31 Root shape design of dental implants. (A) Flat cone plus cylinder. (B) Cone. (C) Wide neck cylinder. (D) Cone plus cylinder. (E) Cylinder. (F) Bullet.

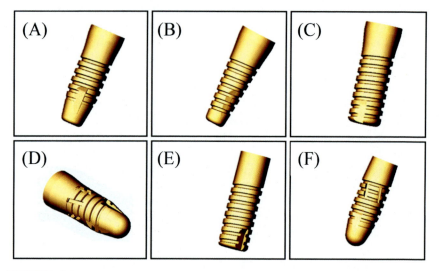

FIGURE 6.32 Antirotation design on the central screw. (A) Antirotation pad on the neck. (B) Pad on column. (C) Double-threaded structure. (D) Surface coating.

5. Antirotation structure on the foundation pile

For the foundation pile, we compared Morse taper matched with the implanting nail by adding the antirotation platform, antirotation edge, and an inner hexagonal structure separately, as seen in Fig. 6.33C. We finally chose the structure of an inner hexagonal

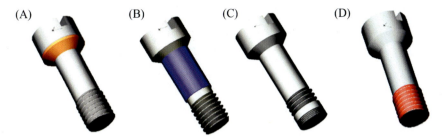

FIGURE 6.33 Antirotation design on the foundation pile. (A) Antirotation shoulder. (B) Antirotation edge. (C) Hexagonal antirotation.

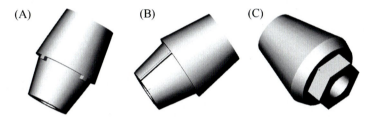

FIGURE 6.34 Accessories for dental implants. (A) Oblique pile. (B) Ball head pile. (C) Healing pile. (D) A transfer. (E) A replaced tool. (F) Repair cap.

platform penetrating the implant and a part of the cone, which can effectively integrate the design requirements of easy processing, matching level, antirotation ability, and sealing degree.
6. Accessories for dental implants

After implantation there is a need to design an oblique pile, spherical pile, and so on to adapt to different practical requirements. A series of accessories are also needed to repair the upper structure, including healing abutments, transfers, replacements, and repair caps, which are shown in Fig. 6.34.

6.5.2 Structural simulation optimization and biomechanical analysis of TLM dental implants

6.5.2.1 The structural optimization of a TLM dental implant

3D modeling software was used for entitative assembly. The obtained assembly of dental implants consisted of threaded implant entity, central screw, and cancellous bone entity. The implant's outer screw threads were required to be fully engaged with the inner screw threads

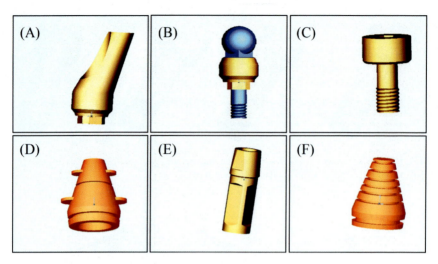

FIGURE 6.35 Structure design of Ti dental implants. (A) 3D model. (B) Model imported into analysis software. (C) Boundary constraints.

of the cancellous bone, and the specific mechanical parameters of materials and load were as follows:

1. Mechanical parameters: The elastic modulus of the cancellous bone was 0.8 GPa, with a Poisson's ratio of 0.3. The elastic modulus of the implant was 103.4 GPa, with a Poisson's ratio of 0.35. The elastic modulus of cortical bone was 13.7 GPa, with a Poisson's ratio of cortical bone of 0.3.
2. Load: The applied torque load was 35 Nm, applied on top of the abutment.
3. Boundary conditions: material setting with continuity, small deformation, cylindrical-type setting for the shape of the implant.

3D modeling software was used to draw a 3D geometrical model of threaded dental implants and localized bone of the lower jawbone. The external conical surface of the upper end of the abutment was applied with a torque of 35 Nm for finite element simulation. CP-Ti and TLM alloy were chosen to fabricate dental implants that were 4.0 mm in diameter, 13.0 mm in length, and 0.8 mm in pitch. The thread section was approximately an obtuse triangle. The upper abutment of the dental implant model was simplified to be a hexagonal cylinder with a diameter of 3 mm and a height of 3 mm. The 3D model calculation of the dental implant is shown in Fig. 6.35. The bone part was 28.6 mm × 25.4 mm × 10 mm, and the inside for cancellous and outer surface for cortical with 1.5 mm in thickness were set. The center of the cancellous bone was designed to

6.5 Implants for oral and maxillofacial repair and replacement of TLM alloy

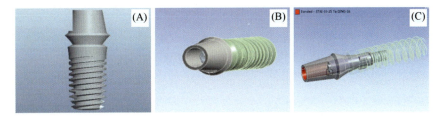

FIGURE 6.36 Structure analysis of implant components. (A) Meshing. (B) Adding the torque.

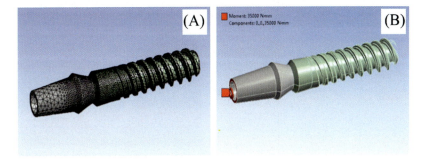

FIGURE 6.37 Stress analysis of Ti dental implant components. (A) Foundation pile. (B) Central screw. (C) Implants.

contain a threaded implant socket, which was fully engaged with the implant thread.

The structure of dental implants was divided into 10-node tetrahedral element SOLID187 and 20-node hexahedral element SOLID186. Meshing is a key factor in finite element analysis. The quality of meshing directly affects the accuracy of the analysis results. We used a fully automatic meshing method, which has good adaptability. In the analysis of linear structural statics, only the properties for Young's modulus, Poisson's ratio, and density of designated material are needed. The mechanical analysis showed that the implant structure needed to be improved and optimized, but the finite element simulation provided quick guidance for the initial structural designing. Details are seen in Figs. 6.36 and 6.37.

6.5.2.2 Biomechanical CAE analysis of a TLM dental implant

The thickness of the neck of the dental implant near the gingival part is reduced, which will form a stress relief ring structure. The stress ring design is helpful to ease the transmission of bite force. The model design and the finite element meshing of a dental implant in simple shape and the bone blocks are shown in Fig. 6.38. A certain bite force

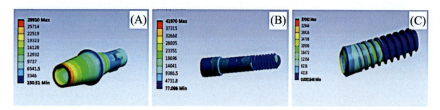

FIGURE 6.38 The finite element model of dental implant and its meshing.

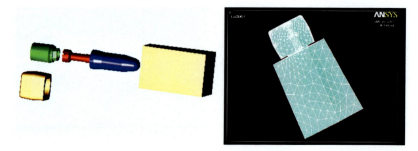

FIGURE 6.39 The stress distribution cloud diagram in a dental implant with a stress relief ring.

that can be decomposed in the directions parallel and perpendicular to the axis of the implant is applied to the upper part of the tooth. All surface displacement of the dental model is fixed. The results of cloud diagram for stress distribution are shown in Fig. 6.39.

The stress curve from the top edge of the implant to its bottom is shown in Fig. 6.40. The stress ring design is located 0–0.5 mm below the top of the implant as shown in Fig. 6.40A. It can be seen that the maximum stress is located at 1–2 mm below the top. In the case of the nonstress ring design, as shown in Fig. 6.40B, the stress gradually decreases, that is, the bite force of the tooth can be transmitted through the dental implant and thus cause a stress shield. By contrast, when there exists a stress ring design as shown in Fig. 6.40A, the stress drops rapidly from the maximum stress point, which effectively reduces the stress-shielding effect and facilitates the formation of new bone.

According to the results of finite element simulation, we invented a variety of novel dental implants [23–26]. These implants were multithreaded spiral implants, which can increase the contact area with the jawbone, reduce bone loss during implantation, improve antirotation performance, and improve postoperative stability. A guiding ball head

6.5 Implants for oral and maxillofacial repair and replacement of TLM alloy

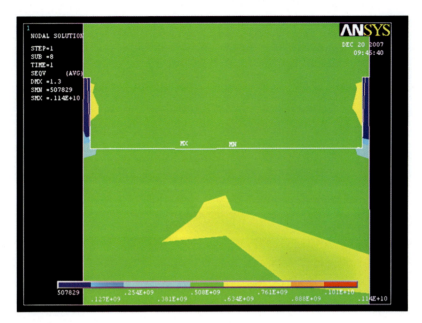

FIGURE 6.40 Stress distribution of dental implants from top to bottom. (A) With the stress ring. (B) Without the stress ring.

TABLE 6.6 Specifications of TLM alloy dental implants.

No. (x: length)	Diameter, D (mm)	Length, L (mm)
S1 − x	3.2	7, 8, 9.5, 11, 12, 14
S2 − x	3.6	7, 8, 9.5, 11, 12, 14
B1 − x	4.5	7, 8, 9.5, 11, 12
B2 − x	5	7, 8, 9.5, 11, 12

was designed at the bottom of the implant, the outer surface was a taper-to-straight external thread, and there were no fewer than two spiral blade grooves on the external thread. The upper end was a polygonal structure, and the center of the implant had a blind hole and an internal thread. The implant was not easy to loosen after being implanted and stable for a long time. The abutment can be fixed at the regular polygonal position of the upper end of the implant by tightening the screw to complete the surgical restoration. Table 6.6 shows the specifications of TLM alloy dental implants determined by our preliminary design, which is shown in Fig. 6.41.

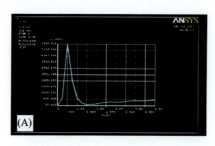
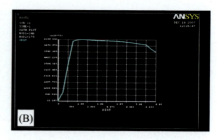

FIGURE 6.41 Photograph of TLM dental implants.

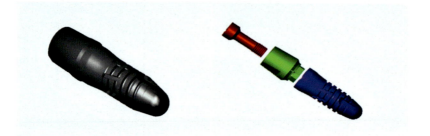

FIGURE 6.42 Photographs of TLM dental implants. (A) after precision machining. (B and C) The surface treated with HA coating. *HA*, Hydroxyapatite.

6.5.3 Precision machining of TLM alloy dental implants

The process route of processing are as follows:

1. Implant
   Ti wire (Φ3–5 mm) → Blanking → Turning (external surface) → Milling (antirotation groove) → Drilling (the clamp) and tapping → Upsetting and extruding (inner hexagonal connecting hole) → Tapping → Turning (outer thread) → Polishing
2. Foundational pile
   Wire (Φ3–5 mm) → Blanking → Turning external shape → Milling → Drilling → Cutting → Surface polishing
3. Central screw
   Wire (Φ3–5 mm) → Blanking → Turning the center screw shape → Turning external thread → Milling grooves → Cutting → Surface treatment

Using the above process, we can machine a variety of TLM alloy dental implants with different structures and different microarc oxidation and polishing treatments to perform surface modification treatments [27,28], which are shown in Fig. 6.42.

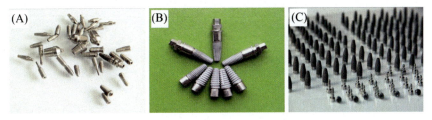

FIGURE 6.43 3D-printed dental samples. (A) Dental implant. (B and C) Laser-printed crown.

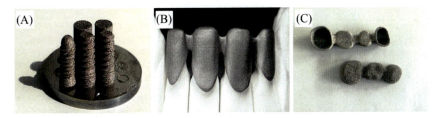

FIGURE 6.44 Spinal fixation system made of TLM alloy. (A) Top view. (B) Side view.

In recent years, on the basis of a large amount of clinical data and CT scan results, we have established a dental implant design model and processed porous TLM alloy dental implants and crown samples through laser rapid prototyping, as shown in Fig. 6.43. Biomechanical and osteogenic analyses were also carried out [29,30].

6.6 Medical devices of TLM alloy for spine repair

6.6.1 Fixation system for spine

The human spine is connected by a large number of parts, including joint vertebrae, intervertebral discs, ligaments, and muscle tissue. Spinal devices are used mainly to repair, replace, or correct spinal bone fractures, deformities, or degenerative diseases. The main products contain spinal internal fixation systems (including straight round rods, mesh rods, joint rods, threaded rods), shaped rods and fusion cages, matching screws, and so on [31–33].

On the basis of the feedback of clinical data and the 3D characteristics of a Chinese skeleton, a spinal fixation system made of TLM alloy was designed and developed, as shown in Fig. 6.44.

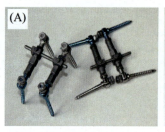 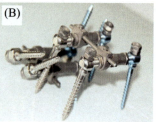

FIGURE 6.45 Medical spine devices made of TLM alloy. (A) Spine cage. (B and C) Porous artificial spine restoration.

6.6.2 Other medical devices made of TLM alloy for spine repair

Thick-walled tubes of TLM alloy 14 mm in diameter and 2 mm in wall thickness were processed for spinal fusion. Two new spine restoration devices made of TLM alloy had also been produced by means of laser powder additive technology, which are shown in Fig. 6.45.

References

[1] Z. Yu, S. Yu, J. Cheng, X. Ma, Development and application of novel biomedical titanium alloy materials, Acta Metallurgica Sinica 53 (2017) 1238–1264.
[2] Q. Chen, G. Thouas, Metallic implant biomaterials, Materials Science and Engineering, R. Reports 87 (2015) 1–57.
[3] Z. Yu, L. Zhou, L. Luo, J. Niu, L. Wang, S. Yuan, et al., Process, microstructure, properties of newly developed β-type biomedical titanium alloy TLM, Chinese Journal of Rare Metals 30 (2006) 226–230.
[4] M. Jackson, J. Kopac, M. Balazic, D. Bombac, M. Brojan, F. Kosel, Titanium and titanium alloy applications in medicine, Surgical Tools and Medical Devices, Springer, 2016, pp. 475–517.
[5] Y. Luo, L. Yang, M. Tian, Application of biomedical-grade titanium alloys in trabecular bone and artificial joints, Biomaterials and Medical Tribology, Elsevier, 2013, pp. 181–216.
[6] F.H.S. Froes, Titanium for medical and dental applications—an introduction, Titanium in Medical and Dental Applications, Elsevier, 2018, pp. 3–21.
[7] F. Ory, J.L. Fraysse, Titanium and titanium alloys: materials, review of processes for orthopedics and a focus on a proprietary approach to producing cannulated bars for screws and nails for trauma, Titanium in Medical & Dental Applications, Elsevier, 2018, pp. 65–91.
[8] P. Gubbi, T. Wojtisek, The Role of Titanium in Implant Dentistry, Titanium in Medical and Dental Applications, Elsevier, 2018, pp. 505–529.
[9] M. Niinomi, Titanium in Medical and Dental Applications | | Titanium Spinal-Fixation Implants, Elsevier, 2018, pp. 347–369.
[10] Van C. Mow, Rik Huiskes, Basic Orthopedic Biomechanics and Mechano-Biology, Shangdong Science & Technology Press, 2009.
[11] A.D. Pye, D.E.A. Lockhart, M.P. Dawson, C.A. Murray, A.J. Smith, A review of dental implants and infection, Journal of Hospital Infection 72 (2009) 104–110.

References

[12] L. Kunčická, R. Kocich, T.C. Lowe, Advances in metals and alloys for joint replacement, Progress in Materials Science 88 (2017) 232–280.

[13] C. Emmelmann, P. Scheinemann, M. Munsch, V. Seyda, Laser additive manufacturing of modified implant surfaces with osseointegrative characteristics, Physics Procedia 12 (2011) 375–384.

[14] B. Yue, K.M. Varadarajan, S. Ai, T. Tang, H.E. Rubash, G. Li, Differences of knee anthropometry between Chinese and white men and women, Journal of Arthroplasty 26 (2011) 124–130.

[15] P. Heinl, L. Müller, C. Körner, R.F. Singer, F.A. Müller, Cellular Ti–6Al–4V structures with interconnected macro porosity for bone implants fabricated by selective electron beam melting, Acta Biomaterialia 4 (2008) 1536–1544.

[16] J. Zhang, W. Bao, Application of minimally invasive technology in traumatology, Guide of China Medicine 11 (2013) 46–47.

[17] M. Geetha, A.K. Singh, R. Asokamani, A.K. Gogia, Ti based biomaterials, the ultimate choice for orthopaedic implants—a review, Progress in Materials Science 54 (2009) 397–425.

[18] Z. Yu, J. Cheng, Y. Zhang, X. Ma, B. Wen, H. Liu, et al., A Test Device With Metal Fatigue and Friction Performance Detection Function, Application Number: CN 201810072348.X.

[19] Q. Chen, H. Guo, K. Avery, X. Su, H. Kang, Fatigue performance and life estimation of automotive adhesive joints using a fracture mechanics approach, Engineering Fracture Mechanics 172 (2017) 73–89.

[20] A.C. Messellek, M.O. Ouali, A. Amrouche, Adaptive finite element simulation of fretting wear and fatigue in a taper junction of modular hip prosthesis, Journal of the Mechanical Behavior of Biomedical Materials 111 (2020) 103993.

[21] Y. Su, S. Yuan, Modern Dental Implantology, People's Medical Publishing House, 2004.

[22] S. Lim, H. Park, S. Lim, H. Choo, S. Baek, H. Hwang, et al., Can we estimate root axis using a 3-dimensional tooth model *via* lingual-surface intraoral scanning? American Journal of Orthodontics and Dentofacial Orthopedics 158 (2020) e99–e109.

[23] S. Yuan, Z. Yu, J. Han, Q. Huangfu, A kind of dental implant, Authorization Number: ZL201210199027.9 (2015).

[24] S. Yuan, Z. Yu, J. Han, Q. Huangfu, A kind of combined dental implant, Authorization Number: ZL201520771839.5 (2016).

[25] S. Yu, Z. Yu, S. Yuan, C. Liu, J. Han, J. Niu, A Kind of Dental Implant With Gradient Porous Structure, Application Number: CN 201610481191.7.

[26] S. Yu, Z. Yu, S. Yuan, J. Han, J. Niu, A Kind of Implantwith Porous Thread Structure for Dental Implant Application Number: CN 201711249959.3.

[27] S. Yuan, Z. Yu, S. Yu, C. Liu, J. Niu, Q. Huangfu, et al., A kind of blind hole polishing device for dental implant, Authorization Number: ZL201210199027.9 (2015).

[28] S. Yu, Z. Yu, J. Niu, C. Liu, J. Han, Y. Zhang, et al., A Method for Preparing Composite Coating on Surface of Titanium Alloy Dental Implant, Authorization Number: CN 201510300936.0.

[29] Y. Zhao, Y. Zhang, Z. Yu, L. Kong, Y. Zhao, Mechanical analysis of titanium alloy with low elastic modulus for ceramic-metal, Rare Metal Materials and Engineering 38 (2009) 1386–1389.

[30] W. Jing, M. Zhang, L. Jin, J. Zhao, Q. Gao, Assessment of osteoinduction using a porous hydroxyapatite coating prepared by micro-arc oxidation on a new titanium alloy, International Journal of Surgery 24 (2015) 51–56.

[31] R.D. Bowles, L.A. Setton, Biomaterials for intervertebral disc regeneration and repair, Biomaterials 129 (2017) 54–67.

[32] N. Kitpanit, S.H. Ellozy, P.H. Connolly, C.J. Agrusa, A.D. Lichtman, D.B. Schneider, Risk factors for spinal cord injury and complications of cerebrospinal fluid drainage in patients undergoing fenestrated and branched endovascular aneurysm repair, Journal of Vascular Surgery 73 (2020) 399−409.

[33] R. Nardone, C. Florea, Y. Höller, F. Brigo, V. Versace, P. Lochner, et al., Rodent, large animal and non-human primate models of spinal cord injury, Zoology 123 (2017) 101−114.

CHAPTER 7

Development and application of TLM alloy for treatment of soft tissue with minimally invasive surgery

7.1 Development and application survey of minimally invasive devices

Titanium (Ti) alloys have been widely used in the repair and replacement of human bones and hard tissues such as artificial joints, spine, limbs, and craniomaxillofacial parts. Since the beginning of the 21st century, with the development of advanced manufacturing technologies in the precision mechanical and electronic industries, Ti and its alloy materials have also been widely used in the manufacturing of interventional and minimally invasive medical devices for the repair and replacement of soft tissues, such as cardiovascular and cerebrovascular tissues, as well as for hemodialysis and other blood contact devices. Especially in the heart, brain, and vascular system, implanted devices have complex mechanical environments and higher comprehensive performance requirements. These devices include heart valves, cardiac occluders, artificial hearts, brain stimulators, and cardiocerebrovascular stents [1]. Devices that are in contact with blood have to be not only able to serve reliably to maintain specific physiological and mechanical functions, but also safe and compatible with the biological environment in which they are located. Thus these devices have especially stringent requirements in terms of comprehensive physical and chemical properties, biological properties, safety, and the structural design and long-term service performance for metal implanting and interventional materials [2].

Compared with traditional surgical implants, implants for minimal access therapy are a large category of passive and active medical devices with small and precise structure design that conduct through percutaneous and human narrow entrances and exits or tracts such as the oral cavity, nasal cavity, anus, or urethra. Because of the minimal trauma and the convenient and flexible process (sometimes requiring interventional endoscopic imaging observation) during surgery, Ti alloy materials, in particular the ultrafine wires that are 50–500 μm in diameter, tubes with smaller diameters (1–3 mm) and wall thicknesses (0.1–0.3 mm) and foils with 10–300 μm thicknesses have great application potential and broad prospects in treating various soft tissue diseases, such as those of the heart, liver, gallbladder, breast, cardiovascular and cerebrovascular systems, and digestive tract.

In the late 1980s the first successful coronary stenting surgery was carried out in the United States. This milestone technology has saved the lives of many patients and has also improved their quality of life. From the earliest bare metal stents to the second-generation drug-eluting stents, the success rate of percutaneous transluminal coronary angioplasty has greatly increased, and the problem of restenosis has been solved to a certain extent [3]. In 2012, Abbott Company of the United States took the lead in launching the bioabsorbable vascular stent. In 2016 the German Biotronik Company also launched the first drug-eluting degradable magnesium alloy stent and obtained European Union and Conformite Europeenne certification. Judging from the current research and development status, the degradable metal stent is being developed on the basis of mature drug-eluting stents [4]. The main aims lie in material innovation, but the safety assessment of long-term restenosis of the stents still needs to be investigated in depth. With the continuous development and progress of minimally invasive interventional therapy technology, its use has been gradually extended to the treatment of other peripheral vascular and nonvascular diseases [5,6]. For example, the TiNi alloy with super elasticity was first used for self-expansion-type coronary vascular stents and then was applied in other nonvascular stents, such as esophageal and biliary stents, owing to their low supporting force and extreme flexibility. Related vascular, nonvascular stents and application fields are shown in Table 7.1.

The world's first buried pacemaker was successfully developed in Sweden in 1958. It has experienced four generations of products since then, which is the only effective way to treat bradycardia, and has saved the lives of countless patients [7]. In the past 20 years, active medical devices have developed rapidly all over the world. Brain pacemaker (Deep Brain Stimulation) is the biggest breakthrough in the treatment of Parkinson's disease. Its working principle is to connect a finer electrode with less than 1 mm in diameter to a microcomputer stimulator the size

TABLE 7.1 The classification of human soft tissue and application in vascular interventional therapy.

Classification of human soft tissues			Application in interventional therapy
Cardiovascular	Peripheral vascular	Nonvascular	
Coronary arteries Intracerebral arteries	Carotid artery Renal artery Thoracoabdominal artery Limb artery Vein artery Iliac artery	Pancreatic duct Esophagus Intestinal canal Biliary tract bronchus Airway Urethra	Cardiology, cardiology, neurology, general internal medicine, oncology, urology, pediatric celiac, obstetrics and gynecology, otolaryngology, etc.

of a matchbox, the former is place it in a specific part of the brain to coordinate the activities of the human body by stimulating the nerve signals that control the human movement in the brain. Ventricular-assisted devices are another epoch-making product that has been a boon for a large number of congestive heart failure patients. The third generation of new compact implantable, magnetic levitation, and centrifugal artificial hearts has now been developed. Its working principle is to use a magnetic levitation centrifugal pump and the connecting catheter to transport blood.

Whether it is a vascular stent or an artificial heart, these high-end products are inseparable from various advanced medical metal materials with thin-walled tubes, foils, and wires, such as stainless steel, cobalt-chromium alloy, Ta refractory metal, PtIr precious metal, and nickel-Ti alloy. Ti alloys, especially β-type Ti alloys, with medium and high strength, low elastic modulus, good plastic toughness, fatigue resistance, and corrosion resistance, are especially easy to process into various plates, rods, wires, tubes, and other materials. they show promise for use in the field of minimally invasive interventional therapy for cardiovascular and cerebrovascular diseases [8].

7.2 Design and manufacture survey of interventional devices

The development and application of metal coronary stents have produced self-expanding stents and balloon-expandable stents. The self-expanding stent utilizes the shape memory effect or superelasticity of the material. The compressed stent is automatically restored to its original shape after being delivered to the diseased part *via* the catheter. TiNi alloy is an ideal material for self-expanding stents and has been widely used in clinical practice [3]. The balloon-expandable stent is delivered through operation of pressing and holding it on the balloon, delivering it to the target lesion with a catheter, expanding the stent through inflation of the balloon, and then withdrawing the balloon and catheter. At present, the balloon-expandable stents that are widely used in clinical practice include 316L stents of medical stainless steel and L605 stents of cobalt-chromium alloy.

The processing and preparation methods of metal vascular stents have successively experienced the development of wire weaving, flat plate photoetching coil welding, and laser etching of thin-walled tubes. The filament braided stent has a simple process and good flexibility but has poor strength, uneven deformation, and a high axial shrinkage rate. It is difficult to ensure the dimensional accuracy of roll-welded stents made *via* thin-plate lithography-photoetching. With the successful development of thin-walled tubes of high-strength TiNi alloy and CoCr alloy, the precision laser-cutting technology has been used to hollow out small-diameter and thin-walled tubes, and this has become the main processing method of coronary stents [8]. Compared with the first two methods, three-dimensional laser processing facilitates the overall structure design, good processing accuracy, and high efficiency with low cost. In the meantime, compared with braided or welded structural stents, stents fabricated directly from tubes have a thinner wall thickness, which is conducive to the unobstructed lumen of the diseased site. The hollow structure of the tubular stent can also be designed to achieve a larger radial expansion ratio and smaller axial contraction. Typical filament braided stents and laser-engraved stents are shown in Figs. 7.1 and 7.2.

Currently, the types of lasers used in vascular stent cutting include CO_2 lasers, Nd:YAG lasers, light fiber lasers, and ultrashort pulse lasers. According to the differences in laser pulse width, they can be divided into long-pulse-width lasers (≥ 10 ps, including CO_2, Nd:YAG, and most light fiber lasers) and ultrashort-pulse-width lasers (≤ 10 ps, such

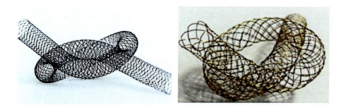

FIGURE 7.1 Two typical wire braided metal stents.

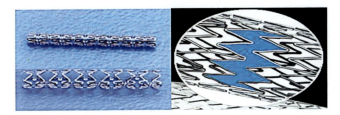

FIGURE 7.2 Two typical laser-engraved stents.

as picosecond and femtosecond lasers). The cutting mechanism of the long-pulse-width laser is to melt or evaporate the material matrix by heat, and blow away the molten material to form a slit under the action of the coaxial airflow of the laser beam. The ultrashort pulse width laser has a very high energy density, and the material can be removed by vaporization in an instant. The main process parameters for laser cutting include laser power, pulse width, frequency, focus position, cutting speed, auxiliary gas and air pressure, etc. The combination of different process parameters can achieve different cutting qualities.

Laser microconnection is also considered to be a better method for the manufacture of metal vascular stents. On one hand, it can realize the small size and complex structure of stents, thereby making possible the interventional treatment of brain microvascular disorders. On the other hand, it can keep the maximum shape memory effect and superelasticity of TiNi alloy. We chose a 500-W pulsed laser to weld Ti50.6% Ni alloy wire that was 0.5 mm in diameter, and the results showed that when small current and large pulse were used, the melting area was composed of dendrites, while the part of the heat-affected zone near the molten pool was coarse equiaxed crystals, and the area near the matrix material was finer equiaxed crystals.

At present, the cases of active medical devices such as artificial hearts and brain stimulators are all made of thinner plates of CP–Ti or Ti6Al4V alloy. The commonly used processing methods are warm stamping (deep drawing) and secondary shaping or being processed by four to five passes of deep drawing, bulging, and shaping at room temperature [9,10]. This puts forward higher requirements for the cold formability, stamping, and bending properties of Ti alloys. During cold rolling or cold drawing, the deforming direction will be more consistent with the increase in the amount of deformation, and a fibrous structure may even form, which leads to the difficulty of secondary redeforming of the alloy, owing to the significant increase of dislocation density. In addition, the Ti alloy may form a cold deformation texture after cold working, leading to the formation of anisotropy [11]. But the superb deep-drawing performance and bending performance of the thinner plates and strips could be improved though the control of different fiber texture structure of Ti alloys.

7.3 Coronary stents of TLM alloy

The research and development of cardiovascular stents is based mainly on the collaborative development of materials in the fields of mechanical engineering, biology, clinical medicine, and iconograph medicine. Therefore researchers in various fields have been working hard to develop ideal novel alloy materials that can be used for intravascular stents, design more reasonable stent structures, and conduct long-term clinical evaluations to achieve the best biocompatibility and mechanical compatibility in order to overcome later coronary thrombosis and restenosis [12]. A comparison of the technical performance of cardiovascular stents developed worldwide is shown in Table 7.2. A large number of clinical results show that stents made of traditional stainless steel, Ti-nickel alloy, and cobalt-chromium alloy all contain

TABLE 7.2 Comparison of technical performance of vascular stents developed worldwide.

Stents Parameter	MAGIC coronary stent	GR II coronary stent	Palmaz-Pchatz coronary stent	Balloon-expandable stent
Ingredient	Core metal Pt, surface layerCoCr alloy	316L stainless steel (nonferromagnetic)	316L stainless steel (nonferromagnetic)	316L (nonferromagnetic)
X-ray visualization	Excellent	Excellent	Moderate	Moderate
Vessel wall covering area	About 14%	Average 16%	Expanded area >80%	Expanded area >80%
Cross-sectional area	0.062 mm^2	–	–	–
Stent shape	Round	Sheet, plate-shaped	Diamond	Diamond
Stent thickness	0.08–0.10 mm	0.127 mm	0.07 mm	0.09 mm
Profile	1.53–1.6 mm	2.5–1.42 mm 3.0–1.52 mm 3.5–1.68 mm 4.0–1.78 mm 4.5–1.80 mm 5.0–1.85 mm	1.5 mm	1.5 mm
Retraction rate after stent expansion	15%–20%	–	2.5%–5.3%	2.5%–13.2%
Effective diameter range	Fully opened4.0–6.0 mm	2.5, 3.0, 3.5, 4.0, 4.5, 5.0 mm	3.0, 3.5, 4.0 mm	3.0, 3.5, 4.0, 5.0 mm
Implant length	15–50 mm	12, 20, 40, 60 mm	15 mm	8, 9, 14, 18 mm
Expansion of device	Self-expanding delivery system	Balloon	Balloon	Balloon
Minimum inner diameter of catheter	1.63 mm	1.47–1.90 mm	2.2 mm	2.2 mm
Cladding tube	Needed	Not needed	Needed	Needed
Recommended expansion pressure	Not needed	4–6 atmospheres	4 atmospheres	6 atmospheres

Co, Cr, and Ni elements, which have harmful effects on the human body. After long-term vascular intervention the precipitation of harmful ions can easily induce serious lesions. Although the application prospects of degradable metal stent materials such as magnesium alloy, zinc alloy, and pure iron are promising, no breakthrough has been made in terms of the controllable degradation rate and the harm caused by the dissolution of a large number of ions into the human body. In recent years, with the continuous in-depth application research into metastable β-Ti alloys with no toxic elements, high strength, and low modulus, the comprehensive properties of the novel TLM alloys developed by the Northwest Institute for Nonferrous Metal Research (NIN) are comparable to those of the CoCr alloy stent materials currently being used in clinical practice. And the TLM alloy makes it easier to produce high-quality small-diameter, thin-walled tubes, which are expected to become an ideal vascular stent material [13]. The mechanical properties and samples of the TLM alloy small-diameter thin-walled tubes (also called capillaries) are shown in Table 7.3 and Fig. 7.3, respectively.

TABLE 7.3 Typical mechanical properties of small-diameter and thin-walled TLM alloy tubes.

Tube size (mm)	R_m (MPa)	R_p (MPa)	A_5 (%)	E (GPa)	Burst pressure (MPa)	Remarks
Φ1.6 × 0.18	1268	1024	12	63.2	360	Cold drawn
Φ2.0 × 0.18	922	808	17	64.9	–	Cold drawn + aging
Φ6.0 × 0.50	630	465	51	75.9	–	Cold rolled + annealing

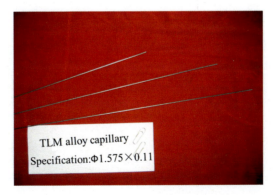

FIGURE 7.3 Tube samples of small-diameter and thin-walled TLM alloy.

7.3.1 Stent pattern selection of TLM alloy

According to the current common vascular stent patterns, by taking into account the coverage area of the stent's vascular wall, radial support strength, flexibility, and other factors, we have determined that the Z-shaped structure of the vascular stent has a large radius of support, good transportability, and good adhesion, which can significantly reduce the retraction rate of the TLM alloy stent, as shown in Table 7.4.

7.3.2 Radial support force of a TLM alloy stent

The novel TLM alloy and 316L stainless steel stent materials were subjected to a compressive load of 1.33 N, and the compressive mechanical properties were compared. The basic parameters of the two alloy materials are shown in Table 7.5 and Fig. 7.4.

TABLE 7.4 Selection and design of a vascular stent of TLM alloy.

Vascular stent pattern	Vascular stent structure and performance prediction
Z-shaped	The serrated closed ring and the axial S-shaped connector are matched and have good support and flexibility. The shrinkage rate and the axial retraction rate are small, and the metal coverage rate is low.
Oval rhombus–shaped	The stent has large radius support strength and good flexibility, easily conforms to the contour of the blood vessel, and has good axial stability.
M-shaped	The support strength of the stent radius is large, the axial retraction rate is less than 3%, and the metal coverage is less than 12%.
Maple leaf–shaped	The stent is uniformly stressed and has good compliance after expansion, and the system is versatile and flexible. The axial retraction rate is ≤2%, and the radial contraction rate is ≤3%.
S-shaped	The stent has high support strength, good flexibility and compliance, and reduced metal coverage.
Bow-shaped	There is strong support in the radius, and the transportability and adhesion are good, which can significantly reduce the retraction rate of the stent.

7.3 Coronary stents of TLM alloy

TABLE 7.5 Basic parameters of TLM alloy and 316L alloy.

Material	E (GPa)	R_p (MPa)	R_m (MPa)
316L	201	280	750
TLM (soft state M1)	42	400	660
TLM (soft state M2)	70	550	860

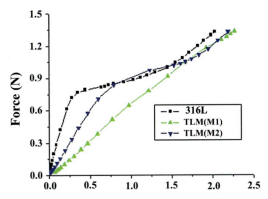

FIGURE 7.4 Compression resistance curve of two alloy materials.

It can be seen from Fig. 7.4 that the two kinds of stents separately made of TLM alloy and 316L stainless steel have similar support performance, and their radial support forces are both greater than 250 g/15 mm, which can meet the practical requirements of vascular stents. The design of any coronary stent should take into account that the stent must be able to easily reach the target blood vessel through the curved coronary artery, so the flexibility of the stents is the main factor for the operation's success. The stent must to be soft and easy to deliver to the lesion and easy to adapt to the shape of the blood vessel and the location of the lesion. Studies have shown that the TLM alloy vascular stent has a lower elastic modulus or stiffness. Therefore the TLM alloy stent has good flexibility in blood vessels, and its longitudinal flexibility is higher than that of other materials, such as 316L stainless steel. On this basis, if TLM alloy is treated by solid solution and aged state, that means that when the tensile strength is controlled above 900 MPa and the Young's modulus is about 80 GPa, the support strength performance of the alloy stent can be further improved while maintaining excellent flexibility [14–16].

7.3.3 Retraction rate test and finite element analysis of a TLM alloy stent

According to calculations, when the diameter of the original small-diameter and thin-walled TLM tube used for a vascular stent is 1.6 mm, the proportion of the coverage area of the metal part is about 24%; when the diameter of the stent is expanded to 4 mm, the proportion of the coverage area of the metal part will be reduced to 16%. We chose TLM alloy and 316L stainless steel stents with original outer diameters of 1.77 mm for the retraction rate tests. Both stents were expanded to 3.20 mm, and then the stent was released, and the stent rebounded by itself. The TLM alloy has a shrinkage rate of less than 10%, which meets the practical requirements of a blood vessel stent, as seen in Table 7.6.

The shrinkage rate of the TLM alloy stent was subjected to finite element numerical simulation. The specific process was as follows:

1. Establish a solid model under Pro/E, including 1/2 stent (middle symmetry), and add two upper and lower rectangular rigid planes and cylindrical rigid support surfaces.
2. Import the built model into ANSYS software.
3. Input the material properties of the stent, including the elastic modulus and plastic deformation curve.
4. The solution is divided into three load steps: the expansion of the stent, the stent's elastic contraction, and the stent's radial compression.
5. After completing the first load step, remove the contact pair between the inner surface of the stent and the support cylinder surface, and release the displacement constraint of the support surface. Then start solving the second load step.
6. After completing the second load step, apply constraints in the UX direction to the lower rectangular surface, and apply a concentrated force of 1.33 N to the upper rectangular surface. Then start the third load step.
7. After completing the third load step, postprocess for the results.

The finite element numerical simulation results are consistent with the measured value of the shrinkage rate, as shown in Fig. 7.5.

TABLE 7.6 Retraction rates of the stents of TLM alloy and 316L.

Stent material	Radial rebound (mm)	Radial rebound rate (%)
316L stainless steel	0.061466	1.918
TLM alloy (soft state M1)	0.183964	5.736

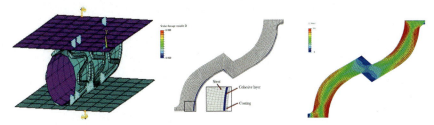

FIGURE 7.5 Finite element analysis of the compression of a TLM alloy vascular stent.

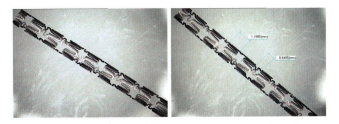

FIGURE 7.6 A TLM alloy stent and its structural dimensions.

7.3.4 Processing and postprocessing of a TLM alloy stent

Combining with the geometrical dimension factors of the small-diameter and thin-walled TLM alloy tube, the ANSYS software finite element simulation is used to complete the analysis and calculation of the length, width, and distribution density of the struts and the bridge of the TLM alloy vascular stent. The specific stent design structure and the size are shown in Fig. 7.6. The stent design is 19 mm in length and has 10 S-shaped bridges in total. Each S-shaped section has 3 S-shaped strut parts and 11 V-shaped strut parts (9 large V-section struts, one small V-section struts at each end) on its circumference, and each large V-section strut has 6 V-section struts on the circumference and 9 small V-section struts on the circumference at the end of stent.

1. Processing of a TLM alloy stent

    The laser-engraving machine is used to precisely cut the small-diameter and thin-walled TLM alloy tube. The specific processing is as follows:

    First, the design optimization and programming of the laser-cutting path of the vascular stent need to be completed, then the corresponding machine language is input, and the path running test is carried out. Secondly, carry out laser (Nd:YAG laser) etching test for TLM alloy tube under argon protection, including laser energy setting, pulse wavelength and spot size, and appropriate moving speed of tube sample, etc. To achieve a complete cutting state and minimize the burrs at the same time, we finally determined the best laser energy (pulse energy) to be 5−20 mJ, the pulse width to be 500−2000 ms, the spot size to be controlled at 1−5, and the proper moving speed to be 5−40 mm s^{-1}. The laser machine and TLM alloy stent cut are shown in Fig. 7.7.

2. Posttreatment of a TLM alloy stent

In the ultrasonic cleaning machine, the dynamic vibration milling process is used to remove the residues of capillary material, burr, and oxidation pollution layer on the surface of the TLM alloy. Through experimental study, the ratio of chemical milling fluid was determined to be industrial common nitrate acid (HNO_3), hydrofluoric acid, corrosion inhibitor, and water (H_2O) at a weight ratio of 8%−12%:1%:2%:82%−86%, respectively. The ultrasonic frequency was 30−50 kHz, and the duration time was 5−15 minutes. The surface quality of the stent blank was improved.

Electrochemical polishing must be done to further brighten the surface of TLM alloy stent. Determining the best electrochemical polishing process is very important to ensure the excellent surface quality and geometrical size of the TLM alloy stent. The process charts of electropolishing are as follows:

Deoiling (derusting) → Ultrasonic cleaning → Pickling → Ultrasonic cleaning → Liquid blending → Polishing liquid cooling → Electrolytic polishing → Water washing → Natural drying

The ratio of solvent for electrochemical polishing determined by experiment is as follows: 3:15:80:1 with 20 mL of perchloric acid, 140 mL of methanol, 240 mL of *n*-butanol, and 8 g of additive, respectively. The experimental temperature is room temperature. The schematic diagram of the electrochemical experimental device and the microscopic morphology of the polished samples are shown in

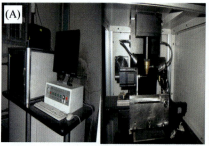
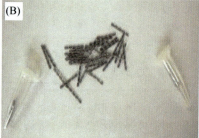

FIGURE 7.7 Processing of TLM alloy stents. (A) Laser-engraving machine. (B) Stent samples.

Fig. 7.8. Table 7.7 shows the parameters of the electrochemical polishing test. Photos of the original and polished stents by laser engraving are shown in Figs. 7.9 and 7.10.

3. Biochemical corrosion performance of a TLM alloy stent

    Sheet samples of 2 mm × 25 mm × 50 mm of TLM alloy were chosen. The surface oxide layer of each sample was removed, and then the samples were soaked in soapy water for 10 minutes, followed by rinsing with tap water, rinsing with distilled water, and drying with filter paper. The corrosion rate (R value, unit: mm y^{-1}) was determined at 60°C and room temperature (20°C–25°C) in 3.5% NaCl aqueous solution by referring to the Method of Uniform

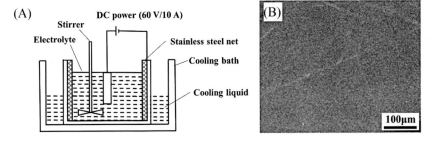

FIGURE 7.8 Electrochemical polishing test. (A) Schematic diagram. (B) Surface scanning morphology of a TLM alloy stent.

TABLE 7.7 Parameters for electrochemical polishing for the TLM alloy stent.

Main electrolyte composition	Voltage (V)	Time (s)	Temperature (°C)
Perchlorate + n-butyl alcohol + methanol	12–18	10–100	30
	17–20	<80	25
	5–25	<120	27
	10–20	<150	25
	5–20	50–130	19

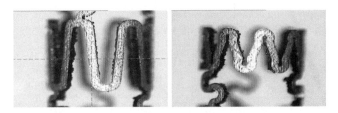

FIGURE 7.9 Original state of a TLM alloy stent by laser etching.

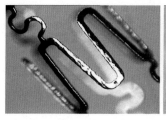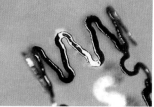

FIGURE 7.10 TLM alloy stents after electrochemical polishing.

Corrosion Total Impregnation Test for Laboratory of Metal Materials (JB/T7091-1999).

Through the above experimental tests, the biochemical corrosion rates of TLM alloy stent are 0.0008 mm y^{-1}, which shows that the TLM alloy has excellent corrosion resistance and can meet the practical requirements of a vascular stent in the human body.

7.4 Nonvascular stents and related devices of TLM alloy

In 1969, Dotter first placed a spring-shaped stent made of stainless steel wire into the artery of a dog and proved that the metal stent could be inserted into a vessel to maintain the patency of the vessel. Since then, the metal stent has been widely used in the clinical treatment of various vascular stenosis. The application of vascular stents in nonvascular stenosis or obstructive lesions has been widely promoted, including those in the esophagus, bile duct, stomach, duodenum, proximal jejunum, nodal (rectus) intestine, bile duct, trachea and main bronchus, prostatic urethra, ureter, and nasolacrimal duct [17,18]. In 1983, Frimberger applied a TiNi alloy stent to treat malignant esophageal stenosis and achieved a good effect of relieving esophageal obstruction. In the same year, China began to use this therapy for treating advanced esophageal cancer stenosis. At that time, the implantation of esophageal stents was mainly carried out under surgical thoracotomy, which was characterized by large trauma, high postoperative complication and mortality rates, and narrow indications. In 1989, Iving reported for the first time that 16 cases of malignant biliary stricture and 9 cases of benign biliary stricture were relieved after implantation of Z-type metal stents. In 1990, Giliams successfully placed a metal mesh stent into the stenosis of the biliary tract through the first percutaneous transhepatic bile duct puncture. In 1993, Zongjun Dong et al. successfully placed a TiNi alloy stent under an endoscope for the treatment of esophageal stenosis or obstructive lesions. In 1994, Renjie Yang et al. first reported the successful placement of self-made self-expanding Z-type stainless steel coated metal stents under X-ray guidance (without endoscope) for the treatment of 14 cases of esophageal cancerous stenosis. In 2010, Dr. Aixing Tan of Xi'an Tangdu Hospital developed a prosthesis for the repair of laryngotracheal defects in cooperation with the author's group [19–21].

7.4.1 Larynx and trachea prosthesis of TLM alloy

TLM alloy sheet (0.5 mm in thickness) was selected and made into a concave microporous thin piece by laser cutting, drilling, and special mold pressing. The overall shape of the throat prosthesis was diamond-like, concave, and 2.0 cm in height, about 20 mm in length, 10 mm in width, 60–80 μm micropore in diameter, and 30%–35% in porosity, as shown in Fig. 7.11.

The TLM alloy prosthesis was cleaned by ultrasound and sterilized by high pressure before implantation. Five standard hybrid (mongrel) dogs weighing 12–15 kg were selected. Fibrolaryngoscopy (Nissan ENF-V2 type) was used to detect the effects during 3–6 months after surgery. All animals were operated on in a modern operating room according to relevant national standards. The postoperative thin-walled larynx prosthesis of TLM alloy was used to repair anterior larynx defect, as shown in Fig. 7.12.

The experiment found that all five dogs in this study survived the operation, with no airway obstruction, prosthesis displacement, or granulation tissue growth on the surface of the lumen. The prosthesis cleavage was observed in all the tested dogs, and all showed good biomechanical strength. A representative beagle dog was selected for nasopharyngoscopy, as shown in Fig. 7.13. The experimental results showed that a small number of secretions remained on the surface of the repaired internal lumen on the third day after surgery (Fig. 7.13A),

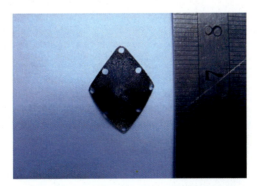

FIGURE 7.11 A thin-walled larynx prosthesis made of TLM alloy. *Source: data from A. Tan, Application and Research of New Meso-Stabilized β-Titanium Alloy in Reconstruction of Larynx and Trachea Defects, Department of Otolaryngology, Tangdu Hospital, Fourth Military Medical University, 2011.*

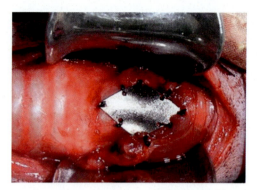

FIGURE 7.12 TLM alloy repair of a defect in the anterior larynx. Source: *data from A. Tan, S. Cheng, P. Cui, P. Gao, Replacement of an anterior larynx split with a β-type titanium alloy prosthesis in subglottic stenosis: a preliminary study in canine, Modern Oncology 12 (2012) 2486-2488.*

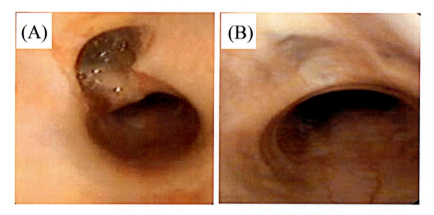

FIGURE 7.13 Morphology of a TLM alloy larynx prosthesis after implantation. (A) Three days after laryngeal reconstruction. (B) Four months after laryngeal reconstruction. Source: *data from A. Tan, S. Cheng, P. Cui, P. Gao, Replacement of an anterior larynx split with a β-type titanium alloy prosthesis in subglottic stenosis: a preliminary study in canine, Modern Oncology 12 (2012) 2486–2488.*

and the edges formed a good combination with the host tissue, without congestion or edema. Four months after implantation, the graft was almost completely fused with the adjacent laryngotracheal tissue, with smooth epithelium visible on the surface of the reconstructed area (Fig. 7.13B). In animal experiments, it was found that the surrounding connective tissue could quickly grow into the airway lumen through the micropores and promote the growth of the epithelium. The TLM alloy laryngeal prosthesis was implanted with satisfactory therapeutic effect.

7.4.2 Laryngeal repair tube-type devices of TLM alloy

We also use laser drilling and microwelding methods to develop a TLM alloy strip into tissue engineering scaffolds with microporous structure, nonvascular lumen scaffolds, and other devices. For example, to realize the vascularization and epithelialization of nonvascular soft tissue lumen as soon as possible, we used laser engraving to prepare tube-type laryngeal repair devices of TLM alloy with micropores. The experimental strip material was 0.5 mm in thickness, and the micropore size was designed to be 40–60 μm, as shown in Fig. 7.14. It can be seen that the micropores on the surface of the laryngeal scaffold processed by laser drilling are evenly distributed, which is conducive to cell adhesion, proliferation, and differentiation; promotes the growth of chondrocytes and long-term stable service *in vivo*; and can also effectively prevent restenosis of the larynx, as shown in Fig. 7.15.

7.4.3 Blood circulation pipe fittings of TLM alloy

Chinese researchers are actively exploring the use of biomedical Ti alloy instead of stainless steel to make pipeline systems for blood

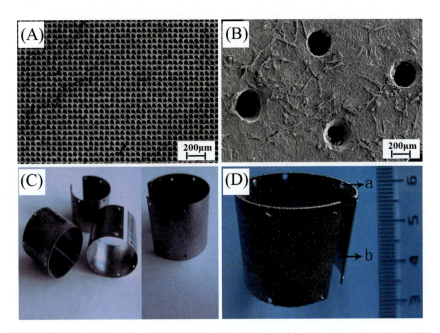

FIGURE 7.14 Some tube-type devices for laryngeal repair made of TLM alloy. (A) and (B) Photos of microporous preforms. (C) and (D) Tube-type samples after rolling. Source: *B and D data from A. Tan, S. Cheng, P. Cui, P. Gao, J. Luo, C. Fang, et al., Experimental study on an airway prosthesis made of a new metastable β-type titanium alloy, The Journal of Thoracic and Cardiovascular Surgery, 141 (2011) 888-894.*

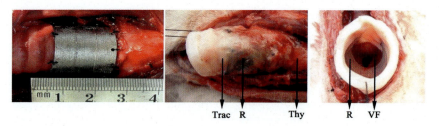

FIGURE 7.15 Animal test of laryngeal repair tube-type devices made of TLM alloy. *Source: Fig. 7.14B and D data from A. Tan, S. Cheng, P. Cui, P. Gao, J. Luo, C. Fang, et al., Experimental study on an airway prosthesis made of a new metastable β-type titanium alloy, The Journal of Thoracic and Cardiovascular Surgery, 141 (2011) 888-894.*

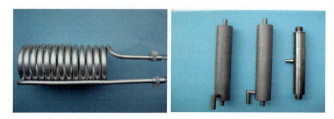

FIGURE 7.16 Piping system of blood filtration made of TLM alloy.

separation or filtration in medical devices or instruments that are in contact with blood, such as heart valves, blood dialyzer, and oxygenators, for which there are very strict requirements on blood compatibility of materials. The bending is a very complicated process of plastic and elastic deformation for Ti alloy tubes (pipes). During the bending deformation the inner part of tube will become be thicker, while the outer will become thinner, and the maximum bending strain occurs on the outermost surface. When the external force is removed, the bending Ti pipes will produce a certain rebound, so that the bending radius and bending angle increase, which will affect the forming accuracy of the bending pipe, even leading to local wrinkling, thinning, flat holes, cracks, and other defects. Because of its good cold working formability and welding performance, TLM alloy can be easily processed into special piping systems for blood separation, filtration, or dialysis equipment [22−24], as shown in Fig. 7.16.

7.5 Shell of brain and heart active devices of TLM alloy

At present, the key component of the cardiac pacemakers on the market is mainly made of CP−Ti and Ti6Al4V alloy thin plates that are

0.3–0.4 mm in thickness [25]. Although CP–Ti has good biocompatibility and is easy to process into plates and strips, its low strength and high modulus are not desirable for this usage, while Ti6Al4V alloy with higher strength and poor cold forming property is also not an ideal material. TLM alloy is wonderful candidate with high strength, low elastic modulus, good plasticity, and easy machining into plates or strips with fine crystallization. By using finite element simulation software (Deform), our research team optimized the stamping process parameters of CP–Ti and TLM sheets, which is 0.4 mm in thickness, and successfully developed the shell-type samples of pacemakers [26–29]. The valuable technical data have been accumulated for the research and development of artificial heart products.

7.5.1 Model establishment

1. Setting preprocessing parameter

    Before simulation we need to set the preprocessing parameters, which are the basic mechanical property parameters of pure Ti sheets obtained by tensile tests at room temperature, as shown in Table 7.8.

    Other parameters can be obtained by referring to relevant literature and materials. The thermal conductivity, heat transfer coefficient, thermal expansion, heat capacity, emissivity, density, and Poisson's ratio of the material are 15.07 W (m K)$^{-1}$, 15.07, 8.2 × 106, 0.126 J (g °C)$^{-1}$, 0.2, 4.54 g cm^{-3}, and 0.3, respectively. Sparse solver and Newton–Raphson iterative methods were used in this simulation to reduce the computation time.

2. Pro/E modeling

    We made use of Pro/E 5.0 software to model the pacemaker shell designed by our group and obtained the upper mold and the lower mold. The blank shape was developed by Pro/E software, and the blank holder was designed according to the shape of the die, as shown in Fig. 7.17.

7.5.2 Influence of process parameters

1. Influence of the average strain rate

    With other parameters unchanged, we studied the influence of different average strain rates on the stamping forming of TA1 CP–Ti shell, as shown in Fig. 7.18. It can be clearly seen from the figure that

TABLE 7.8 The mechanical property parameters CP–Ti sheet.

Plate thickness (mm)	R_p (MPa)	R_m (MPa)	A (%)	E (GPa)
0.4	262	364	46	102.7

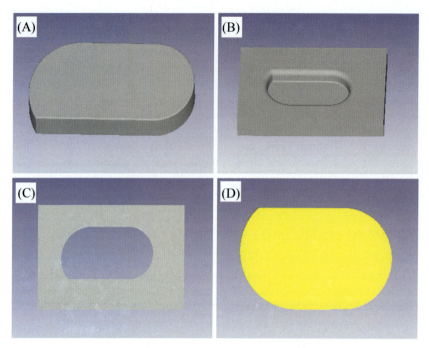

FIGURE 7.17 Die modeling design of a CP−Ti shell. (A) Top of die. (B) Bottom of die. (C) Blank workpiece. (D) Blank holder. *Source: data from J. Shi, B. Wen, Z. Yu, J. Cheng, Study on plastic forming of the cardiac pacemaker outer shell based on DEFPRM, Journal of Plasticity Engineering 24 (2017) 81-86.*

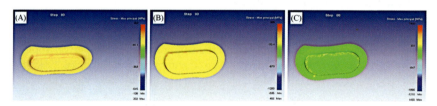

FIGURE 7.18 Maximum principal stress cloud images with different average strain rates. (A) 1×10^{-4} s^{-1}. (B) 1×10^{-3} s^{-1}. (C) 1×10^{-2} s^{-1}.

as the average strain rate increases, the maximum principal stress on the shell part increases exponentially, indicating that the forming becomes more and more difficult.

2. Influence of friction factors

    In the process of stamping, three main aspects are involved in friction: friction between punch and sheet material (friction coefficient set as μ_1) and friction between die, blank holder, and sheet material (friction coefficient set as μ_2). As can be seen in Fig. 7.19, with the increase of

7.5 Shell of brain and heart active devices of TLM alloy

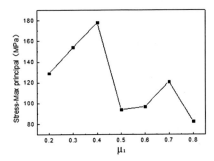 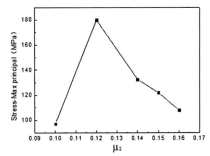

FIGURE 7.19 Effect of μ_1 and μ_2 on the maximum principal stress of a CP–Ti plate.

friction coefficient μ_1, the maximum principal stress on shell part presents a trend of increase, decrease, increase, decrease. The smaller the maximum principal stress, the less easy it is for the sheet metal to crack and the more favorable it is for stamping on the sheet. But the value of μ_1 cannot be too large; it means that the punch surface is very rough and it will cause scratches on the sheet surface. Therefore in the actual processing, it is necessary to consider comprehensively according to the processing requirements, and the μ_1 value selected in this experiment is most appropriate at 0.5–0.6.

It has also been found that the maximum principal stress increases first and then decreases with the increase in μ_2. We think that the optimal value of μ_2 is 0.1, which can greatly improve the slip between blank holder, die, and sheet metal and is beneficial to improve the stamping formability on the Ti sheet.

3. Influence of unilateral clearance between the punch and the die

The clearance between the punch and the die has a great influence on sheet stamping deformation. If the clearance is too large, the side wall of sheet metal easily become curved, or the profile of the shell may become a cone with a small bottom and big mouth. If the gap is too small, it is easy to make the side wall of the sheet thin, and even the phenomenon of cracking may appear. In addition, if the clearance is too small, it will make the contact pressure between the die surface and the sheet material increase, and the abrasion on the die will also increase. Fig. 7.20 shows the influence of the clearance between the punch and the dies on the maximum principal stress. As can be seen, the maximum principal stress decreases with the increase in clearance and 0.4 mm in minimum value. The smaller the clearance, the greater the maximum principal stress, which indicates that the contact pressure between the material and the die indeed increases, resulting in flow difficulty of the material. Thus from the finite element simulation

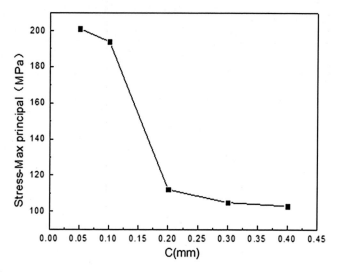

FIGURE 7.20 Effect of the clearance between the punch and the die on the maximum principal stress.

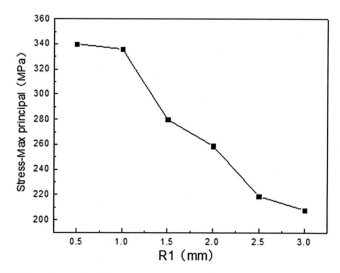

FIGURE 7.21 Effect of the fillet radius of the bottom die on the maximum principal stress.

and analysis we determined that the optimized single side clearance is 0.4 mm.

4. The influence of die fillet radius

Fig. 7.21 shows the effect of different die fillet radii r_1 on the maximum principal stress in the stamping. It can be seen from the figure that the maximum principal stress decreases gradually with the increase in the die fillet radius r_1, indicating that the larger the die fillet radius is, the easier the material flow will be and the more conducive to stamping. Compared with that of 3 mm in fillet radius, when the r_1 value is set 0.5 mm, the maximum principal stress increases about 1.6 times. By means of numerical simulation we determined that an r_1 value of 3 mm is most appropriate.

Through the numerical simulation of pure Ti shell stamping process under the above different parameters, the influence of different parameters on the stamping performance of Ti and its alloy sheet can be studied. According to the basic mechanical properties of different Ti materials, we should try to improve the maximum forming ability of the sheet as much as possible and reduce the residual stress and the rebound it caused at the same time [27,28]. Fig. 7.22 shows the springback simulation analysis of stamping forming of Ti alloy shell parts for a cardiocerebral pacemaker. The optimal process parameters for stamping of pure Ti TA1 sheet are shown in Table 7.9.

The cases of active medical devices, such as cardiac pacemakers, artificial auxiliary hearts, and brain stimulators, are generally formed of parts with large depth and complex profile. By using the above-mentioned numerical simulation method and specific industrial experiment verification, we successfully developed a TLM alloy case for a cardiac pacemaker, an artificial assisted heart, and others, as shown in Fig. 7.23.

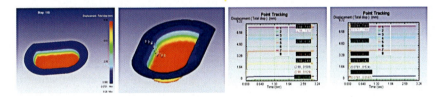

FIGURE 7.22 Springback simulation analysis of stamping of CP–Ti shell parts for a pacemaker.

TABLE 7.9 Optimum process parameter for Ti shell stamping.

Process parameters	Recommended values
Mean strain rate (s^{-1})	1×10^{-4}
Friction (μ_1)	$\mu_1 = 0.5-0.6$
Friction (μ_2)	0.1
Single side clearance between punch and die (mm)	0.4
Rounded radius of die (mm)	3

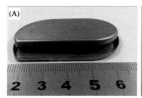 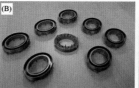 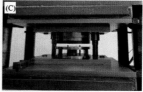

FIGURE 7.23 Photos of some typical TLM alloy cases and related stamping equipment. (A) Case of artificial auxiliary heart. (B) Intestinal stapler. (C) 100-t press.

7.6 Other minimally invasive and interventional devices of TLM alloy

In 2003 our research team at NIN successfully developed a new type of near-β biomedical Ti alloy TLM, and we have obtained several Chinese national invention patents [28–31]. The novel material contains a certain proportion of zirconium, molybdenum, niobium, and tin elements, which are beneficial to the human soft and hard tissue. TLM alloy has excellent biocompatibility and mechanical properties, including a low modulus, high strength, high plasticity and toughness, and a high fatigue limit, by which their comprehensive mechanical properties are broadly adjustable and can be matched according to different applications in nearly all kinds of medical devices under different process and heat treatments. In particular, TLM alloy has excellent cold and hot deformation workability and a wide processing window and thus results in a simple and efficient process and lower cost. At present, a variety of industrial raw materials are produced with the traditional pressure processing equipment, including plates, rods, tubes, strips, and forgings. In particular, the wires (50 μm in smallest diameter), capillary tubes (1 mm in smallest diameter, 0.1 mm in smallest wall thickness), and foils (20 μm in smallest thickness) were also successfully produced, and more than 10 enterprises standards were established. The typical materials are shown in Figs. 7.24 and 7.25.

TLM alloy not only possesses a wide range of wonderful mechanical properties, but also has certain functional characteristics, such as superelasticity and a shape memory effect, so it can meet the special design and application requirements of different surgical implanting and interventional devices [1,2], as shown in Fig. 7.26.

In recent years, with the continuous improvement of medical technology, along with the rapid development of new advanced manufacturing technologies, precision machinery and electronic industries, those medical devices, especially in cutting-edge fields, such as active medical devices and minimally invasive interventional medical devices endowed with multifunction capabilities, intelligent, miniaturization, lightweight, portable, as

FIGURE 7.24 Ultrafine wires of TLM alloy. (A) Wire samples. (B) Finer crystal microstructure. (C) Ultrafine wires.

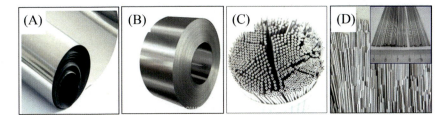

FIGURE 7.25 Foil and capillary tubes of TLM alloy. (A) and (B) Foil samples. (C) and (D) Capillary tubes in longitudinal and transverse directions.

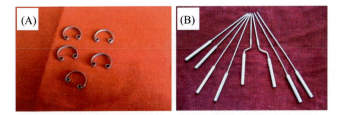

FIGURE 7.26 TLM alloy medical devices. (A) Cochlear prosthesis. (B) Surgical tools.

well as new concepts, new methods and new technologies, have been becoming the key and important development trends and directions in the future [2]. We believe that there are wider application prospects for novel TLM alloy materials in the near future.

Reference

[1] Z. Yu, L. Zhou, X. He, L. Luo, L. Liu, Development and application of titanium alloy materials for human hard tissue repair and replacement, Journal of Functional Biomaterials 37 (2006) 664–670.
[2] Z. Yu, S. Yu, J. Cheng, X. Ma, Development and application of novel biomedical titanium alloy materials, Acta Metallurgica Sinica 53 (2017) 1238–1264.

[3] Z. Zhao, D. Liu, Y. Zhang, Research progresses in endovascular stent biomaterials, Chinese Journal of Medical Instrumentation 29 (2005) 391–395.
[4] F. Huang, S. Yuan, J. Han, Z. Yu, S. Yu, Y. Zhang, et al., Advance in biodegradable stent, Materials China 34 (2015) 396–400.
[5] F. Huang, S. Yuan, Z. Yu, J. Han, J. Cheng, Y. Zhang, et al., Biodegradable magnesium alloy tubes and biliary stent, Guangzhou Chemical Industry 43 (2015) 54–56.
[6] C. Wang, Z. Yu, Y. Cui, Y. Zhang, S. Yu, G. Qu, et al., Processing of a novel Zn alloy micro-tube for biodegradable vascular stent application, Journal of Materials Science and Technology 32 (2016) 925–929.
[7] J. Shi, B. Wen, Z. Yu, Y. Cui, Y. Zhang, L. Wang, et al., Recent progress and development trend of cardiac pacemaker, Biomedical Engineering and Clinical Medicine 20 (2016) 639–645.
[8] Z. Yu, L. Zhou, F. Huang, S. Yuan, Y. Zhang, J. Niu, et al., R & D and application on Ti alloy capillary material used in vessel intervention, China Medical Device Information 12 (2006) 15–20.
[9] C. Yang, Y. Ma, H. Wang, Numerical simulations of automobile sump forming process, Machine Building and Automation 37 (2008) 52–54.
[10] Y. Shang, X. He, Analysis of forming technology and die design for shell parts, Rare Metal Materials and Engineering 01 (2003) 23–24, 35.
[11] Z. Yu, L. Zhou, J. Deng, H. Gu, Investigation on textures of the alloy Ti-2Al-2.5Zr tube and sheet, Rare Metal Materials and Engineering 29 (2000) 86–89.
[12] Y. Zhang, D. Kent, G. Wang, D. St John, M. Dargusch, Evolution of the microstructure and mechanical properties during fabrication of mini-tubes from a biomedical β-titanium alloy, Journal of the Mechanical Behavior of Biomedical Materials 42 (2015) 207–218.
[13] Z. Yu, L. Zhou, G. Wang, Q. Hong, B. Zhao, J. Niu, et al., β-Type titanium alloy for vascular stent, Authorization Number: ZL03153138.5 (2005).
[14] Q. Huangfu, Z. Yu, J. Han, S. Yuan, S. Yu, Z. Yafeng, et al., Research of Ti3Mo2Sn3Zr25Nb alloy for stent, Materials China 35 (2016) 386–390.
[15] Y. Tian, Z. Yu, J. Han, S. Yu, Q. Huangfu, Performance evaluation of TLM titanium alloy for cardiovascular stent application, Biomedical Engineering and Clinical Medicine 17 (2013) 616–620.
[16] Q. Huangfu, Z. Yu, L. Luo, J. Niu, Y. Zhang, X. He, New high strength titanium alloy stent preparation and performance research, Chinese Journal of Rare Metals 30 (2006) 125–128.
[17] Y. Zheng, L. Zhao, Biomedical Nickel-Titanium Alloys, Science Press, 2004.
[18] Z. Yu, M. Zhang, S. Yu, C. Liu, B. Wen, Y. Zhang, Analysis of R&D, production and application of biomedical Ti alloys materials applied in medical devices of China, China Medical Device Information 18 (2012) 1–8.
[19] A. Tan, Application and Research of New Meso-Stabilized β-Titanium Alloy in Reconstruction of Larynx and Trachea Defects, Department of Otolaryngology, Tangdu Hospital, Fourth Military Medical University, 2011.
[20] S. Cheng, C. Liu, Z. Yu, A. Tan, P. Cui, J. Luo, et al., A medical larynx and tracheal stent, Authorization Number: ZL201020289830.8 (2011).
[21] C. Liu, Z. Yu, S. Yuan, S. Yu, J. Han, J. Niu, et al., A preparation method of titanium or titanium alloy laryngo-tracheal interventional stent, Authorization number: ZL 201210543703.X (2015).
[22] S. Yuan, Z. Yu, J. Han, H. Liu, Q. Huangfu, X. Ma, Technical research on small-radius bends of thin-walled capillary tube made from a new β-type titanium alloy, Chinese Journal of Rare Metals 34 (2010) 668–672.

[23] S. Yuan, Z. Yu, C. Liu, S. Yu, Q. Huangfu, Y. Zhang, A Processing Device for Thin-Walled Metal Bending Pipe of Fine Diameter, Authorization Number: CN, 2009 10023968.5.
[24] Q. Shen, S. Yu, J. Niu, B. Wen, S. Liu, Z. Yu, Research progress of implanting fine metal wires and its heterogeneous materials welding technology, Materials Review 33 (2019) 2127−2132.
[25] J. Shi, B. Wen, Z. Yu, J. Cheng, Study on plastic forming of the cardiac pacemaker outer shell based on DEFORM, Journal of Plasticity Engineering 24 (2019) 81−86.
[26] J. Shi, B. Wen, Z. Yu, Y. Cui, Y. Zhang, L. Wang, Influencing factors of titanium and titanium alloys shell's stamp forming and its application status, Titanium Industry Progress 33 (2016) 1−5.
[27] H. Xue, Z. Yu, J. Cheng, J. Niu, S. Yu, W. Zhang, Research status of the stamping of titanium and titanium alloy sheet, Chinese Materials Science Technology and Equipment 11 (2015) 66−68.
[28] B. Wen, Z. Yu, S. Yu, J. Niu, Y. Zhang, X. Ma, et al., The Invention Relates to a Sealing Surgical Stamping Die for Heart and Brain Pacemaker, Application Number: CN 201810610163.X.
[29] S. Yuan, Z. Yu, J. Han, Z. Yu, Q. Huangfu, A single flow nasal suction device, Authorization Number: ZL201420356068.9 (2014).
[30] J. Niu, Y. Gao, Z. Yu, X. Guo, S. Yuan, Minimally invasive orthopedic support plate for funnel chest, Authorization Number: ZL200720033095.2 (2008).
[31] S. Yu, Z. Yu, S. Yuan, C. Liu, J. Niu, Y. Zhang, Titanium alloy guide wire for surgical interventional therapy, Authorization Number: ZL201310682015.6 (2016).

Index

Note: Page numbers followed by "*f*" and "*t*" refer to figures and tables, respectively.

A

Acupuncture materials, 11–12
Albumin, self-assembly of, 150
Alloy dental implants, precision machining of, 194–195, 194*f*, 195*f*
Anodic oxidation, TiO$_2$ nanotube bioactive film preparation, 142–144, 143*f*
Antibacterial stainless steels, 4
Anticoagulant coatings on, 148–153
  albumin, self-assembly of, 150
  composite coatings
    blood compatibility, characterization of, 151–153, 151*t*
    surface characterization of, 150–151, 151*f*, 152*f*
  heparin, self-assembly of, 150
  TiO$_2$ films, preparation and activation of, 149–150
Anticoagulant surface modification, for cardiovascular stents, 130–132
Antimicrobial coatings, 153–159
  phase characterization of, 154–155, 155*f*
  preparation of, 154–155, 155*f*
  properties, characterization of, 157–159, 158*f*, 159*f*
  surface morphology, characterization of, 155–157, 156*f*
AuAgCu alloy composition, 12*t*

B

Barium titanate bioactive coatings, by microarc oxidation, 141, 142*f*
β-type Ti alloys
  design and physical metallurgy of, 27
  composition design, 35*t*, 36*t*
  mechanical properties, 38*t*
  melting, 39–41
  overview, 34–39
  TiNb alloys, 44, 45*f*
  TiNbTaZr alloys, 43
  TiTa alloys, 41–43, 42*f*, 43*f*
  TiZr alloys, 44, 44*t*

TLM alloys. *See* TLM alloys
heat treatment of, 55–56, 57*t*
Bioactive coatings, by microarc oxidation, 137–144
  barium titanate bioactive coatings, 141, 142*f*
  porous bioactive coatings, 137–140, 138*f*, 139*f*, 139*t*
  strontium-containing bioactive coatings, 140, 141*f*
  TiO$_2$ nanotube bioactive film preparation, by anodic oxidation, 142–144, 143*f*
Bioactive metal modification, for bones/teeth hard tissues repairing, 128–130
Biological corrosion behavior, 91, 92*t*
Biomechanical compatibility, of TLM alloys, 109–123
  biomechanical match, 110–111, 110*t*, 111*t*, 112*f*, 112*t*
  conception, 109–110
  dynamic fracture toughness, 120, 120*t*
  grain refinement, 112–113, 113*f*
  high-cycle fatigue deforming performance, 117–118, 118*f*
  low-cycle fatigue deforming performance, 118–120, 119*f*
  phase transformation, 110–111, 110*t*, 111*t*, 112*f*, 112*t*
  shape memory capability, 115–117, 116*f*, 116*t*, 117*f*
  strength and toughness, match of, 112–113, 113*f*
  superelasticity, 113–115, 114*f*, 115*f*
  wearability, 120–123, 121*f*, 121*t*, 122*f*, 123*f*
Biomechanical match, 110–111, 110*t*, 111*t*, 112*f*, 112*t*
Biomedical metal materials
  antibacterial stainless steels, 4
  application of, 4–5
  CoCr alloys, 5–8

228 Index

Biomedical metal materials (*Continued*)
  application of, 8, 9*f*
  mechanical properties of, 6, 7*t*
  microstructure of, 6–8
  overview of, 5–6
  properties of, 6–8
  degradable metals, 19–24
    magnesium alloys, 20–22, 22*f*, 23*f*
    properties of, 21*t*
    zinc alloys, 23–24, 23*f*
  nickel-free austenitic stainless steels, 3, 3*t*
  noble metals, 11–13
    acupuncture materials, 11–12
    AuAgCu alloy composition, 12*t*
    dental materials, 11
    medicinal precious metals, 12–13
    surgical materials, 13
  refractory metals, 13–17
    overview of, 13–14
    porous tantalum application, 16–17, 16*f*
    porous tantalum, preparation and evaluation of, 14–15, 15*f*
  shape memory alloys, 9–10
    brand of, 9–10
    composition of, 9–10, 10*t*
    NiTi shape memory alloys, application of, 10
    overview of, 9
  stainless steels, 1–3
  Ti alloys, 17–19
    applications of, 20*t*
    first generation of, 17–18
    second generation of, 18
    third generation of, 18–19
Biomedical stainless steels, 1–3, 2*t*
Blood circulation pipe fittings, 215–216, 216*f*
Bone plates
  design of, 171–172, 172*f*
  forging, processing and pretreatment for, 172

C
Chemical vapor deposition (CVD), 125–126
Chronic toxicity, 96–102, 100*t*, 101*t*, 102*f*, 102*t*
CoCr alloys, 5–8
  application of, 8, 9*f*
  mechanical properties of, 6, 7*t*
  microstructure of, 6–8
  overview of, 5–6
  properties of, 6–8

Cold rolled tube, of TLM alloys, 73, 73*t*
Coronary stents
  of TLM alloy, 204–212, 205*f*
    finite element analysis, 208, 209*f*
    pattern selection, 206, 206*t*
    processing and postprocessing, 209–212, 209*f*, 210*f*, 211*f*, 211*t*, 212*f*
    radial support force, 206–207, 207*f*, 207*t*
    retraction rate test, 208, 208*t*
    small-diameter and thin-walled tubes, mechanical properties of, 205*t*
    technical performance, 204*t*
Corrosion resistance, 146–148, 147*f*, 148*f*, 149*f*
CVD. *See* Chemical vapor deposition (CVD)
Cytotoxicity, 93–94, 95*t*, 96*f*, 96*t*

D
Degradable metals, 19–24
  magnesium alloys, 20–22, 22*f*, 23*f*
  properties of, 21*t*
  zinc alloys, 23–24, 23*f*
d-electron theory, for Ti alloy design, 28–31, 28*f*, 29*t*, 30*f*, 30*t*
Dental implants
  alloy, precision machining of, 194–195, 194*f*, 195*f*
  biomechanical CAE analysis of, 191–193, 192*f*, 193*f*, 193*t*, 194*f*
  structural design of, 186–189, 186*f*, 187*f*, 188*f*, 189*f*
  structural optimization of, 189–191, 190*f*, 191*f*
Dental materials, 11
Designed hip joint prosthesis
  biotribological analysis of, 179–183, 183*f*
  mechanical simulation of, 178–179, 178*f*, 179*f*, 179*t*, 180*f*
  dynamic, 179–183, 180*f*, 181*f*, 182*f*
Dynamic fracture toughness, 120, 120*t*

E
EBM. *See* Electron beam melting (EBM)
Electron beam melting (EBM), 39, 40*t*
Electroslag remelting (ESR), 39, 40*t*
ESR. *See* Electroslag remelting (ESR)

F
Femoral stem
  design of TLM, 176–177, 177*f*
  manufacture process of, 183–184, 184*f*, 185*f*

Index

G
Genotoxicity, 95–96, 97t, 98t, 99f
Grain refinement, 112–113, 113f

H
Hemolysis, 91–93, 93t, 94f
Heparin, self-assembly of, 150
High-cycle fatigue deforming performance, 117–118, 118f
High-nitrogen nickel-free (HNNF) stainless steel, 3
  mechanical properties of, 3t
HNNF. *See* High-nitrogen nickel-free (HNNF) stainless steel
Hot extrusion tube, of TLM alloys, 72–73, 72f, 73t
Hot forging simulation, 172–174, 173f, 174f, 175f

I
Interventional devices
  design of, 201–203, 202f, 203f
  manufacture survey of, 201–203
Intradermal reaction, 105–106, 106f, 107t

J
Joint repair and replacement, Ti implants for, 174–184, 176f
  designed hip joint prosthesis
    biotribological analysis of, 179–183, 183f
    dynamic mechanical simulation of, 179–183, 180f, 181f, 182f
    mechanical simulation of, 177f, 178–179, 178f, 179f, 179t, 180f
  femoral stem
    design of TLM, 176–177, 177f
    manufacture process of, 183–184, 184f, 185f

L
Laryngeal repair tube-type devices, 215, 215f, 216f
Larynx prosthesis, 213–214, 213f, 214f
Low-cycle fatigue deforming performance, 118–120, 119f

M
Magnesium alloys, 20–22, 22f, 23f
MAO. *See* Microarc oxidation (MAO)
Medicinal precious metals, 12–13
Microarc oxidation (MAO)
  bioactive coatings by, 137–144
    barium titanate bioactive coatings, 141, 142f
    porous bioactive coatings, 137–140, 138f, 139f, 139t
    strontium-containing bioactive coatings, 140, 141f
    TiO_2 nanotube bioactive film preparation, by anodic oxidation, 142–144, 143f
Minimally invasive devices
  application survey of, 199–201, 201t
  development of, 199–201
Mo equivalent, for Ti alloy design, 31–32, 32t

N
Nickel-free austenitic stainless steels, 3, 3t
NiTi shape memory alloys, application of, 10
Noble metals, 11–13
  acupuncture materials, 11–12
  AuAgCu alloy composition, 12t
  dental materials, 11
  medicinal precious metals, 12–13
  surgical materials, 13

O
Oral and maxillofacial repair and replacement, 185–195
  alloy dental implants, precision machining of, 194–195, 194f, 195f
  dental implant
    biomechanical CAE analysis of, 191–193, 192f, 193f, 193t, 194f
    structural design of, 186–189, 186f, 187f, 188f, 189f
    structural optimization of, 189–191, 190f, 191f
Oral irritation, 103–105, 105t, 106f
Orthopedics/trauma repair, Ti implants for, 170–174
  bone plates, design of, 171–172, 172f
  forging of bone plates, processing and pretreatment for, 172
  hot forging simulation, 172–174, 173f, 174f, 175f

P
PBM. *See* Plasma beam melting (PBM)
Phase transformation, 110–111, 110t, 111t, 112f, 112t

230 Index

Plasma beam melting (PBM), 39, 40t
Porous bioactive coatings, by microarc oxidation, 137–140, 138f, 139f, 139t
Porous tantalum
  application of, 16–17, 16f
  evaluation of, 14–15, 15f
  preparation of, 14–15, 15f
Porous titanium alloy, preparation methods and characteristics of, 168t

R
Refractory metals, 13–17
  overview of, 13–14
  porous tantalum, 14–15, 15f
    application of, 16–17, 16f
    evaluation of, 14–15, 15f
    preparation of, 14–15, 15f

S
Shape memory alloys, 9–10
  brand of, 9–10
  composition of, 9–10, 10t
  NiTi shape memory alloys, application of, 10
  overview of, 9
Shape memory capability, 115–117, 116f, 116t, 117f
Skin sensitization and irritation, 103, 103t, 104f, 104t
SMAT. See Surface mechanical attrition treatment (SMAT)
Spine repair, medical devices of TLM alloy for, 195–196
  fixation system, 195, 195f
  porous artificial spine restoration, 196, 196f
  spine cage, 196, 196f
Stainless steels
  antibacterial, 4
  biomedical, 1–3
  nickel-free austenitic, 3, 3t
Strontium-containing bioactive coatings, by microarc oxidation, 140, 141f
Superelasticity, 113–115, 114f, 115f
Surface dealloying, 134–136, 135f, 136f
Surface functionalization, 128–134
  anticoagulant surface modification, for cardiovascular stents, 130–132
  bioactive metal modification, for bones/teeth hard tissues repairing, 128–130
  wear-resistant surface metal modification, for hard tissue replacement, 132–134
Surface hardening modification, 145–146, 145f, 146f
Surface hardness, 146–148, 147f, 148f, 149f
Surface mechanical attrition treatment (SMAT), 144
Surface modification, 125–127
Surgical materials, 13

T
Ti alloys, 17–19
  applications of, 20t
  design of
    β-type. See β-type Ti alloys, design and physical metallurgy of
    composition design, 32–34, 33t
    d-electron theory, 28–31, 28f, 29t, 30f, 30t
    Mo equivalent, 31–32, 32t
    overview, 27–32
  first generation of, 17–18
  surface functionalization of, 128–134
    anticoagulant surface modification, for cardiovascular stents, 130–132
    bioactive metal modification, for bones/teeth hard tissues repairing, 128–130
    wear-resistant surface metal modification, for hard tissue replacement, 132–134
  second generation of, 18
  surface modification of, 125–127, 128f
  third generation of, 18–19
Ti implants
  design and novel manufacture of, 165–170, 166t, 168t, 169f, 170f, 170t, 171f
  for joint repair and replacement, 174–184, 176f
    designed hip joint prosthesis, biotribological analysis of, 179–183, 183f
    designed hip joint prosthesis, dynamic mechanical simulation of, 179–183, 180f, 181f, 182f
    designed hip joint prosthesis, mechanical simulation of, 177f, 178–179, 178f, 179f, 179t, 180f
    femoral stem design, 176–177, 176f, 177f

femoral stem, manufacture process of, 183–184, 184f, 185f
TiNb alloys, 44, 45f
  for orthopedics and trauma repair, 170–174
    bone plates, design of, 171–172, 172f
    forging of bone plates, processing and pretreatment for, 172
    hot forging simulation, 172–174, 173f, 174f, 175f
    traditional, development and application of, 163–165, 164t
TiNbTaZr alloys, 43
TiO$_2$ films, preparation and activation of, 149–150
TiO$_2$ nanotube bioactive film preparation, by anodic oxidation, 142–144, 143f
TiTa alloys, 41–43, 42f, 43f
TiZr alloys, 44, 44t
TLM alloys, 45–51
  anticoagulant coatings on, 148–153
    albumin, self-assembly of, 150
    blood compatibility of composite coatings, characterization of, 151–153, 151t
    composite coatings, surface characterization of, 150–151, 151f, 152f
    heparin, self-assembly of, 150
    TiO$_2$ films, preparation and activation of, 149–150
  antimicrobial coatings on, 153–159
    phase characterization of, 154–155, 155f
    preparation of, 154–155, 155f
    properties, characterization of, 157–159, 158f, 159f
    surface morphology, characterization of, 155–157, 156f
  bars and rods of, 65–71, 66f, 66t, 67f, 67t, 68f, 69f, 70t, 71f, 71t
  billets and semifinished products of, 56–58, 58f, 59f
  bioactive coatings, by microarc oxidation, 137–144
    barium titanate bioactive coatings, 141, 142f
    porous bioactive coatings, 137–140, 138f, 139f, 139t
    strontium-containing bioactive coatings, 140, 141f
    TiO$_2$ nanotube bioactive film preparation, by anodic oxidation, 142–144, 143f
  biological evaluation of, 91–109
    biological corrosion behavior, 91, 92t
    chronic toxicity, 96–102, 100t, 101t, 102f, 102t
    cytotoxicity, 93–94, 95t, 96f, 96t
    genotoxicity, 95–96, 97t, 98t, 99f
    hemolysis, 91–93, 93t, 94f
    intradermal reaction, 105–106, 106f, 107t
    oral irritation, 103–105, 105t, 106f
    skin sensitization and irritation, 103, 103t, 104f, 104t
    subcutaneous, muscle, and bone implantation, 106–109, 108f, 109f
  biomechanical compatibility of, 109–123
    biomechanical match, 110–111, 110t, 111t, 112f, 112t
    conception, 109–110
    dynamic fracture toughness, 120, 120t
    grain refinement, 112–113, 113f
    high-cycle fatigue deforming performance, 117–118, 118f
    low-cycle fatigue deforming performance, 118–120, 119f
    phase transformation, 110–111, 110t, 111t, 112f, 112t
    shape memory capability, 115–117, 116f, 116t, 117f
    strength and toughness, match of, 112–113, 113f
    superelasticity, 113–115, 114f, 115f
    wearability, 120–123, 121f, 121t, 122f, 123f
  coronary stents of, 204–212, 205f
    finite element analysis, 208, 209f
    pattern selection, 206, 206t
    processing and postprocessing, 209–212, 209f, 210f, 211f, 211t, 212f
    radial support force, 206–207, 207f, 207t
    retraction rate test, 208, 208t
    small-diameter and thin-walled tubes, mechanical properties of, 205t
    technical performance, 204t
  design of, 45–46, 46t
  foils, 83–88
    by novel SPD process, 86–88, 86f, 87f, 87t, 88f

TLM alloys (*Continued*)
  SPD processing technology, 83–86, 85*t*
  minimally invasive and interventional devices of, 222–223, 223*f*
  nonvascular stents and related devices of, 212–216
    blood circulation pipe fittings, 215–216, 216*f*
    laryngeal repair tube-type devices, 215, 215*f*, 216*f*
    larynx and trachea prosthesis, 213–214, 213*f*, 214*f*
  for oral and maxillofacial repair and replacement, 185–195
    alloy dental implants, precision machining of, 194–195, 194*f*, 195*f*
    dental implant, biomechanical CAE analysis of, 191–193, 192*f*, 193*f*, 193*t*, 194*f*
    dental implant, structural design of, 186–189, 186*f*, 187*f*, 188*f*, 189*f*
    dental implant, structural optimization of, 189–191, 190*f*, 191*f*
  smelting of, 47–51
  plates and strips of, 58–64, 60*f*, 60*t*, 61*f*, 62*f*, 63*f*, 64*f*, 65*f*, 65*t*
  physical metallurgical properties of, 47–51, 48*t*, 49*f*, 50*f*, 50*t*
  products with special specifications, 77–82
    alloy wires, 82, 83*f*, 84*f*, 84*t*
    small diameters and thin walls, 78–81, 79*f*, 79*t*, 80*f*, 80*t*, 81*f*
    thin walls and variable diameters, 81, 82*f*
  shell of brain and heart active devices of, 216–221
    model establishment, 217, 217*t*, 218*f*
    process parameters, influence of, 217–221, 218*f*, 219*f*, 220*f*, 221*f*, 221*t*, 222*f*
  for spine repair, medical devices of, 195–196
    fixation system, 195, 195*f*
    porous artificial spine restoration, 196, 196*f*
    spine cage, 196, 196*f*
  surface dealloying of, 134–136, 135*f*, 136*f*
  tubes of, 71–77
    cold rolled tube, 73, 73*t*
    hot extrusion tube, 72–73, 72*f*, 73*t*
    relationship among processing, microstructure, and properties, 74–77, 74*f*, 75*f*, 76*f*, 77*f*, 78*f*
  wear-resistant coatings on, 144–148
    corrosion resistance, 146–148, 147*f*, 148*f*, 149*f*
    surface hardening modification, 145–146, 145*f*, 146*f*
    surface hardness, 146–148, 147*f*, 148*f*, 149*f*
Trachea prosthesis, 213–214, 213*f*, 214*f*

V

Vacuum arc remelting (VAR), 39–41, 40*t*, 43
Vacuum induction melting (VIM), 39
Vacuum nonconsumed arc remelting (VNAR), 39, 40*t*
VAR. *See* Vacuum arc remelting (VAR)
VIM. *See* Vacuum induction melting (VIM)
VNAR. *See* Vacuum nonconsumed arc remelting (VNAR)

W

Wearability, 120–123, 121*f*, 121*t*, 122*f*, 123*f*
Wear-resistant coatings on, 144–148
  corrosion resistance, 146–148, 147*f*, 148*f*, 149*f*
  surface hardening modification, 145–146, 145*f*, 146*f*
  surface hardness, 146–148, 147*f*, 148*f*, 149*f*
Wear-resistant surface metal modification, for hard tissue replacement, 132–134

Z

Zinc alloys, 23–24, 23*f*